Exposure Science

Exposure Science
Basic Principles and Applications

Paul Lioy

Clifford Weisel

AMSTERDAM • BOSTON • HEIDELBERG • LONDON
NEW YORK • OXFORD • PARIS • SAN DIEGO
SAN FRANCISCO • SINGAPORE • SYDNEY • TOKYO

Academic Press is an imprint of Elsevier

Academic Press is an imprint of Elsevier
32 Jamestown Road, London NW1 7BY, UK
The Boulevard, Langford Lane, Kidlington, Oxford, OX5 1GB, UK
Radarweg 29, PO Box 211, 1000 AE Amsterdam, The Netherlands
225 Wyman Street, Waltham, MA 02451, USA
525 B Street, Suite 1900, San Diego, CA 92101-4495, USA

First published 2014

British Library Cataloguing-in-Publication Data
A catalogue record for this book is available from the British Library

Library of Congress Cataloging-in-Publication Data
A catalog record for this book is available from the Library of Congress

ISBN: 978-0-12-420167-5

For information on all Academic Press publications
visit our website at **store.elsevier.com**

This book has been manufactured using Print On Demand technology. Each copy is produced to
order and is limited to black ink. The online version of this book will show color figures where
appropriate.

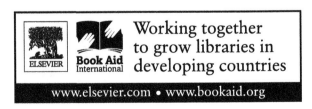

Working together
to grow libraries in
developing countries

www.elsevier.com • www.bookaid.org

DEDICATION

We dedicate this book to the young scientists who will be selecting the study of exposure field as a career path. May their work provide opportunities for solving acute or chronic environmental health problems or preventing exposures that can lead to new problems or unintended consequences in the future.

CONTENTS

ACKNOWLEDGMENTS

The authors wish to thank the members of the field of exposure science for their time, effort and wisdom in bringing substance and recognition to many areas of inquiry now considered part of Exposure Science. We especially want to recognize the efforts of Wayne Ott and Lance Wallace who were true pioneers. There are many, many more individuals that we should recognize, but we would be adding a chapter to this primer on modern exposure science. Personally, Paul would like to thank a few colleagues who have helped make his journey interesting: Drs. Bernard Goldstein (U. Pittsburgh, Emeritus), Edo Pellizzari (Research Triangle Institute, NC, Retired), Phillip Landrigan (Mount Sinai School of Medicine), and Michael Gochfeld (Rutgers U. Robert Wood Johnson Medical School). Finally family, especially my wife Professor Mary Jean Yonone Lioy, who have been there every step of the way. Personally, Cliff would like to thank the many colleagues who helped him develop his understanding of this new and evolving field, in particular Panos Georgopoulos (Rutgers U. Robert Wood Johnson Medical School) and Natalie Freeman (Deceased) and lastly the understanding and encouragement of my family, my wife Fern, children Rachel, Mordecai, and Adam, and my parents, Jack and Claire. We also wish to acknowledge the efforts of Mrs Teresa Boutillette, Mrs Heather Beckles, and Ms Linda Everett in helping to prepare this manuscript.

INTRODUCTION

This book provides the reader with an understanding of the origins and basic principles of human exposure sciences, provides example applications, and defines its utility to both occupational and environmental health. Determination of a person's or a population's exposure is essential for characterizing risks and understanding exposure response—outcome relationships. However, implementation of the concepts and tools of the field has been a challenge [1]. Applications of the basic principles are used to examine contact with a toxic biological, chemical, or physical agent. Within the book, we also describe some fundamental study designs and the types of measurements and associated data needed to characterize human exposure. Since Exposure Science is a relatively new field, we will define its place with respect to other scientific disciplines within the fields of occupational and environmental health. We will present the discussion in a manner that will reduce confusion that still exists about the field. The current confusion was pointed out in a 2013 commentary by Brunekreef who stated that the "latest strategic plan of the International Society of Exposure Science contained nothing but lofty goals and no definitions of Exposure Science and Exposure" [2]. This was based on his observation that dictionaries had different definitions and there were at least 13 attributes ascribed to exposure by professionals in the field, which leads to confusion about the coherence within the field. Thus, after a review of the literature, we offer to the reader a definition of exposure and exposure science that helps refocus discussion on the basic principles of the field [3–6]. In addition to discussions on the tools available for measurement and modeling exposure approaches, we discuss the need to examine the types of human behaviors and activities that significantly influence the types and intensity of contacts that lead to exposure. We expect that the reader will be given a solid foundation in the principles of the field and the methods used to address intensity and duration of human exposures.

REFERENCES

[1] NRC. Exposure science in the 21st century: a vision and a strategy. Washington, DC: The National Academies Press; 2012.

[2] Brunekreef B. Exposure science, the Exposome, and Public Health. Environ Mol Mutagen 2013;54:596–8.

[3] Barr DB. Human exposure science: a field of growing importance. J Exposure Sci Environ Epidemiol 2006;16:473.

[4] Ott WR. Human exposure assessment: the birth of a new science. J Exposure Anal Environ Epidemiol 1995;5:449–72.

[5] Lioy PJ. Assessing total human exposure to contaminants. A multidisciplinary approach. Environ Sci Technol 1990;24:938–45.

[6] Lioy PJ. Exposure science: a view of the past and milestones for the future. Environ Health Perspect 2010;118:1081–90.

CHAPTER 1

History and Foundations of Exposure Science

The origins of the field can be traced to the procedures and measurements used in the fields of occupational and industrial hygiene and radiological health. Some of the first written thoughts about human exposure to toxic agents were presented by Bernardino Ramazzini in his eighteenth century treatise, De Morbis Artificum Diatriba (Disease of the Trades) [1]. As a physician, his focus was on identifying the diseases of workers but at the same time he qualitatively characterized the sources of exposure to the workers and suggested simple ways to prevent such exposures. His efforts and insights were truly ahead of their time, and he remained largely unacknowledged for at least a century. Ramazzini used observation as his primary tool, which is still a very important component of exposure science today. He indicated that in occupational settings simple controls, such as better natural ventilation and reduction in the duration of work tasks can dramatically reduce "contacts" with hazardous agents. Even today adverse health outcomes from exposure to toxicants are often first observed in occupational situations. In particular, some small businesses give little thought to controlling exposure associated with large volumes of toxic agents that are used in their industries. However, in contrast to the historical situations, today more complex controls and strategies are often required to reduce contact and exposure experienced by workers and the general public. In all of the above situations, it should be noted that definitive quantitative knowledge of the severity and frequency of actual health outcomes is not necessarily needed to mitigate, interdict, or prevent exposures to toxic agents.

There are historical examples of environmental situations where effective action was taken prior to complete characterization of the exposure. A classic is based upon the observations of another physician, John Snow, during the 1854 Cholera epidemic. He noted that the high incidence of the disease was occurring among people using water from a well at Broad Street, Soho, near Golden Square. His arguments directly supported work he published 5 years earlier. Snow was able to get the parish (community) to remove the pump handle, disabling the contaminated well thereby reducing exposure to cholera bacteria prior to its biological classification and the incidence of diseases. His ideas were not largely accepted at the time. However, it is another example of the application of exposure science principles to interdict and prevent more disease [2]. By the end of the century, sanitary engineers began to provide systems that separated the sewage system from the water supply system. This pre-environmental management approach effectively eliminated an exposure pathway for microbes thereby preventing waterborne exposures that could lead to disease.

Meaningful advances in the field of occupational hygiene came in the early twentieth century. These were due in part to the pioneering work of Dr. Alice Hamilton who was appointed as head of the Occupational Disease Commission of Illinois in 1908. The position was the first of its kind. The growth of that field over the rest of the twentieth century was summarized by Robert Harris [3]. He pointed out that the first occupational health limits, defined as threshold limit values (TLVs), were published by the American Conference of Governmental Industrial Hygienists (ACGIH) less than 75 years ago in 1945. The Formation of Occupational Safety and Health Administration (OSHA) in the United States in 1971 led to the adoption of formal Occupational Exposure standards called permissible exposure limits (PELs) [4]. Actually, radiation protection standards began to be developed during the early part of the twentieth century and evolved to tolerance limits during World War II. Radiation dosimeters (e.g., film badges) became commonplace by the 1950s and could be considered the first personal exposure monitors. At the same time, biological monitoring for radiation was also used to evaluate exposures and health effects [5,6]. Biological monitoring in other occupational settings started to occur routinely in the 1980s and coincided with the publication of the biological exposure indices (BEIs) by the ACGIH [7].

In 1970, Clean Air Act Amendments legislation were enacted by the US Congress and signed into law by President Nixon. It led to the formation of the US Environmental Protection Agency (USEPA) [8]. The USEPA was charged with addressing and solving environmental pollution problems. The agency developed regulatory standards, control strategies, and mandated the development of enhanced environmental monitoring programs throughout the country for pollutants in the outdoor air, water supplies, and soil. These are used to evaluate compliance with standards and to assess long-term trends in pollution. Other countries have or are starting similar national monitoring programs, and standards or guidelines. Initially, the measurement of exposure *was not part* of the process used to establish the link between pollution concentration and health outcomes to achieve a standard. The emphasis was on measurements of environmental quality. No clear scientific rationale was given for why environmental monitoring rather than exposure characterization was used to develop standards; however, the network siting selections were designed to be population based [9]. The air pollutants initially selected by the USEPA, known as criteria pollutants, and had National Ambient Air Quality Standards (NAAQS) were ozone (photochemical oxidants), total suspended particulate matter, nitrogen dioxide, sulfur dioxide, hydrocarbons, and carbon monoxide. Other pollutants of concern to human health were directly emitted from a variety of sources and were subsequently labeled hazardous air pollutants (HAPs) but without having a specific regulatory standard. Additional pollutants could be considered as surrogates of source emissions or precursors of secondary reactions, e.g., hydrocarbons. Unfortunately, the use of criteria pollutants to represent air pollution left a large gap in our knowledge about the intensity and duration of contact with other airborne toxic agents. The United States and other countries slowly began to measure toxic agents in the air which did not have NAAQS but had water quality standards. These included benzene, toluene, and trichloroethylene. In 1978, lead was added to the list of criteria pollutants and eventually hydrocarbons were delisted as NAAQS.

To provide a context for the problem of using environmental quality data versus exposure data to assess the potential for human health effects, we can look at the EPA Criteria Documents for air pollutants. These are used to provide the scientific basis for the decisions made on the level and form of the NAAQS, but did not include a chapter on exposure until the 1990s. Rather, the original volumes only had chapters on emissions, air quality measurements, toxicology, and health outcomes [10].

Over time this mistake was corrected, but the lack of exposure characterization has not been rectified in monitoring programs. In recent years, more emphasis has been placed on measuring "hot spots" of air pollution which is closer to the susceptible or sensitive population at risk, but the network still primarily reflects compliance with environmental standards and trends.

Historically, major efforts have been made to control outdoor air, water, and soil pollutants, by emphasizing pollutants with large volume emissions rather than understanding their potential for resulting in significant human exposures. In the United States and Europe, however, by the late 1970s, one of these exposure issues was identified—indoor air pollution. Some of the toxicants were relatively unique to indoor sources, e.g., tobacco smoke, but others were exactly the same as those released by outdoor sources. For instance, nitrogen oxides are products of high-temperature combustion of nitrogen in air by oxygen and emitted both indoors and outdoors. The indoor air pollution issue was further complicated during the 1970s because of two energy crises which led to increased use of insulation and reduced ventilation in homes and businesses. One unintended consequence of the expanded use of insulation products and lower ventilation rates indoors in the United States was the introduction of chemicals, e.g., formaldehyde into enclosed structures, which can cause acute health problems. The occurrence of adverse health problems due to being in one's home resulted in some of the first efforts to complete systematic reviews of the problem, including the National Research Council (NRC) report on Indoor Air Pollution [11]. Spengler, Samet, and McCarthy wrote a comprehensive treatise on the indoor air issue which included significant chapters on exposure to many agents, e.g., formaldehyde, nitrogen oxides, radon, and asbestos [12].

At the same time, scientists began to confront the issue of a person's total exposure to individual pollutants and attempted to design programs which could help establish true exposure–response relationships [13,14]. The first comprehensive study to address this issue was the Total Exposure Assessment Methodology (TEAM) project which started in the early 1980s [15–17]. The TEAM study was designed to test various approaches for assessing human exposure. It also attempted to quantify the contributions of outdoor sources of air toxics to total exposure. The most important discovery was that for a variety of toxicants, the main exposures were associated with indoor sources and personal choices about home product use and their storage.

The issue of total exposure was also a source of concern for potable water supplies, both well water and municipal water supplies.

Initially the issues of contaminant exposure from water were focused on drinking the water. However, inhalation and dermal exposures from showering and bathing were identified as a major exposure route for chloroform formed during chlorination of water [18]. Thus, public health directives to not drink the water were changed to: just do not use the water laden with contaminants. During the same period, hazardous waste contamination and removal were estimated by "screening level exposures." A reasonable idea, but this resulted in overestimation of the potential exposure and risk since some point estimates of exposure led to absurd scenarios about how people spent their personal time around such sites. Some of the analyses suggested that people would live on uncontrolled and un-remediated sites for 70 years after detection of the waste. This was a setback in the development of the field of exposure science because it ignored peoples' actual behavior and exposures they experienced. The analyses were subsequently improved when the USEPA developed Monte Carlo methods for calculating better population estimates of exposure. To provide a resource for the field on activities of people that could lead to exposure and provide inputs for the population exposure estimates, the EPA developed an exposure factors handbook which has evolved into an important tool for examining the influence of human factors and activities on exposure [19−22].

1.1 A CONTINUUM FROM SOURCE TO EFFECT: THE ROLE OF EXPOSURE SCIENCE

Exposure science's role in advancing public health can be described as the scientific bridge between environmental science and other disciplines within environmental health sciences. The latter encompasses determination of hazards in laboratory using animals or cell culture (toxicology), and evaluation of human exposure−response relationships (epidemiologic or clinical studies). We have provided a graphic representation, Figure 1.1, of a continuum from source to effects which has been modified or adapted several times since the late 1980s [23−25]. The evolution of Figure 1.1 reflects the maturation of the field as new tools and the principles have been developed within exposure science. The concepts from other versions of the continuum that have been proposed over the years are folded into Figure 1.1 [25−28]. The continuum can be easily transformed to represent occupational situations by renaming its left side: the occupational workplace, and its right side: occupational health sciences.

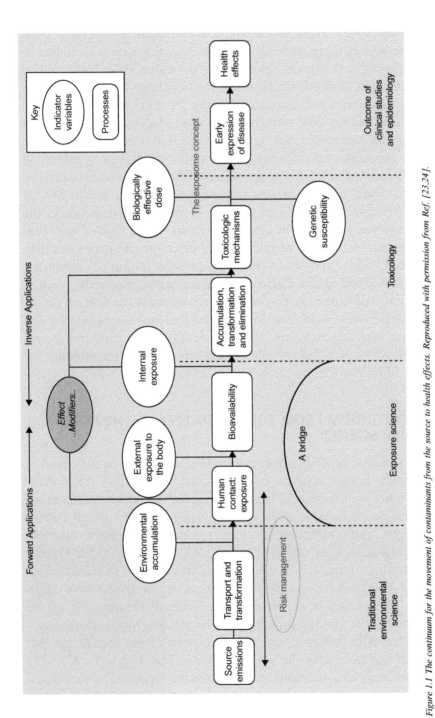

Figure 1.1 The continuum for the movement of contaminants from the source to health effects. Reproduced with permission from Ref. [23,24].

The need for exposure science to act as a bridge is based upon historical research boundaries of traditional environmental science which describes the source of the toxicant, the processes that release it, transform it, and transport it through one or more media (air, water, soil, or food). These areas of inquiry are illustrated on the left side of Figure 1.1. Traditional environmental health sciences describe the processes that occur as a biologically effective dose has been received in the body as depicted on the right side of Figure 1.1. These latter activities include the mechanistic research in toxicology and the human health outcomes examined using epidemiology or clinical practice. Neither side of the continuum directly addresses the fundamental issue of whether and how a human being actually makes "contact" with releases into the environment or workplace. This is addressed by exposure scientists, and the results provide the bridge between these two areas of inquiry. Defining human contact with environmental or occupational agents provides the basis for combining the duration and amount of a toxic agent that can cause a health outcome. Thus, it is essential to link pollutant sources to the behaviors and activities of the human receptor that can result in contact. Exposure science can be used to complete research or applications focused on prevention of exposure and in forensic applications.

Implementation of the exposure science principles and applications as a distinct field has not been recognized until recently. This is because some environmental quality measurements were successfully used as a surrogate for exposure in situations when: (1) once the toxic agent got into an environmental medium it reached the human body or, (2) environmental measurements actually represented a situation that led to significant "contact" with a toxicant by inhalation, ingestion, and/or dermal route. These situations stemmed from the basic fact that in the 1960s and early 1970s the ambient pollution levels were high in air, water, and soil in the United States and other developed countries (e.g., England), and in some cases very visible as gray or orange smog or brilliant sheens on water or soil. As a result, just as in the days of Ramazzini, the identification of high exposures could be obtained from qualitative or quantitative indicators. However, with the introduction of new products and chemicals, and regulations that reduced the frequency of visible ambient pollution levels, it has become essential to develop approaches to properly characterize and classify exposures. At the same time, research on toxicological mechanisms has identified adverse effects at much lower concentrations than previously thought, e.g., lead, arsenic, ozone, and fine particulate matter, as well as identifying the impact of new toxic pollutants released in multiple environments. Thus, the need still exists to address each component of the continuum to help define causes of exposure and the exposure concentrations that eventually affect the body. The continuum, Figure 1.1, is bidirectional. Thus, representative data collected from the right or left side of the continuum can be used as the starting point. The evaluation still passes through the middle and requires an understanding that "contact" has occurred or can occur over a biologically plausible period of time.

From the environmental health perspective, once a toxicant reaches the body, it will be absorbed or adsorbed, and may eventually yield a biologically effective dose [29]. When focusing on the measurements associated with the right side of the continuum, the left side of the continuum cannot be ignored because the biological measurements alone can lead to serious misclassification of the route of exposure and poor characterization of the source of concern. In limited circumstances, events that can lead to a clear relationship between exposure and effects are easily identified and characterized, e.g., chlorine released from a tank car, or an oil slick on a body of water.

One approach used to document that an exposure has occurred is to measure a chemical or metabolite in the body that was associated with an exposure. These measurements are called biomarkers. The place and role of biomarkers in exposure science and environmental health has been a topic of discussion since the CDC issued its first national report card on the levels of toxicants found in bodily fluids in the 1990s as part of the National Health and Nutritional Examination Survey (NHANES) [30]. The NHANES continues to provide an excellent set of biomarker data over time, which is being used to examine the trends in internal exposures to over 100 chemicals. Similar programs are being established in individual states and around the world [30]. The key issue is that we do live in a "chemical world," and the toxic agents we are exposed to can enter our body. They may not, however, be at levels that are a health concern; but, when they are, e.g., lead in blood or organophosphate pesticide metabolites in urine; we will still require the identification of the source and the determination of the important exposure pathways and routes to subsequently mitigate exposure and thereby protect the public health. Thus, as shown in Figure 1.1, a risk management strategy can be developed to determine how best to reduce or eliminate contaminants associated with one or more exposure routes.

The questions raised by people and the press that review the CDC biomarker summaries are: What is causing the exposure, and, if significant, how do we reduce it? Thus, linking the biomarker levels measured to a risk management scheme requires the collection of information on external measurements of exposure, e.g., personal or population monitoring, on activity and behavior pattern data. Characterization or mitigation of job-related exposures of concern is usually more straightforward since workers can wear personal protective equipment (PPE), and/or an industry can substitute a less toxic agent, or add process ventilation. These are not practical for protecting the general public, except in extreme circumstances where PPE can be used for a limited period time.

Mitigation in environmental setting is accomplished by eliminating or reducing the source emissions or secondary products, changing product formulations, or altering people's activities/habits identified by using the principles of the field as in Figure 1.1. Exposure science methodologies should also be required during mitigation to provide information that can be used to educate the public about the situation.

The desire to establish cause and effect relationships between a toxic agent and human health has been a quest of scientific inquiry for many years. As stated above, these have usually started with an observed effect or observed symptoms of a more serious health effect in occupational settings where exposures are high and led to inquiries about the reasons why. Throughout the twentieth century, the inquiries were, in many instances, driven by toxicological research on new or old chemicals used in commerce. The work completed by government, industry, and academia dealt with cause and effect relationships and mechanisms of action using primarily animal models and now "in vitro" techniques. At best they can be extrapolated to "humans," but in many cases are left to describe the hazard. The term hazard can be interpreted as defining the risk in the absence of quantifying the exposure. At best, hazard provides an incomplete assessment of risk. The need for exposure characterization to reduce risks is still one of the two fundamental components for risk assessment and should be subsequently employed to provide effective risk management.

1.2 REGULATION AND EXPOSURE

To better understand workplace occupational exposure assessment, during the mid-twentieth century, personal monitors and room air monitors were developed for toxic gases and particles. The ACGIH began and continues to publish annually the TLVs for many toxic substances emitted into the workplace air, which provides a voluntary effort for controlling workplace exposures to toxic substances [7]. The TLVs are developed using the available toxicological data, and the values are updated based on new toxicological research and workplace-related epidemiologic studies. TLVs have been used as a basis for establishing the PELs used by the Occupational and Safety Health Administration (OSHA) as US workplace standards [4]. Clearly, exposure characterization or assessments are part of the entire effort, but at most were considered an applied science or engineering called industrial hygiene. This was reasonable since many of the problems encountered were primarily associated with very high levels of individual toxicants found in the workplace. As time went on the standards and guidelines began to consider the impact of toxicants on vulnerable worker populations, e.g., women of child-bearing age.

Short of material elimination or replacement of a toxicant, the controls used to reduce exposure included two very important concepts: ventilation, and PPE, respiratory (i.e., respirators) or body (e.g., gloves) protection. Each is employed to reduce "contact" with contaminants in the workplace. However, in industries that produced lead and asbestos, the toxic agent was brought home on clothes, etc. by the workers. The agent could then be contacted by a spouse or children via multiple routes of entry into the body potentially leading to serious health outcomes.

The enactment of the Clean Air Act, Clean Water Act, Occupational Health and Safety Act, and the Mining Safety Act in the 1970s resulted in the development and implementation of federal regulations to control both occupational and community environment emissions of toxicants. There are various regulations associated with each act, as well as additions and revision to laws on the release of toxicants into the environment and their cleanup. These included the Comprehensive Environmental Response, Compensation, and Liability Act (CERCLA) to control or remediate hazardous wastes from sites distributed across the country, and the identification and designation of superfund sites.

The EPA and OSHA enforce the laws associated with each act, and they or other agencies conduct or fund the research necessary to support the laws. Although adequate for the criteria pollutants, i.e., those

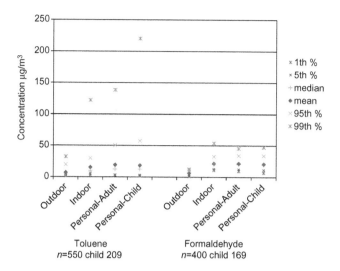

Figure 1.2 Comparison of personal, indoor and outdoor concentrations for toluene and formaldehyde based on New Jersey data from the RIOPA Study.

having EPA NAAQS, in specific outdoor situations ambient air moni-toring as stated above is inadequate for addressing total human contact and exposures [8]. We are still struggling with the lack of comprehensive regulation of products used by consumers or air pollution in the indoor environment which can result in the highest exposures occurring while indoors or due to personal activities, (Figure 1.2). The Consumer Product Safety Commission (CPSC) attempts to deal with exposures related to Consumer Products, and the Food and Drug Administration (FDA) controls the allowable levels of toxicants found in food. For example, unvented or inadequately vented stoves and other combustion sources used indoors for heating can result in higher indoor and expo-sure levels of carbon monoxide (CO) than permitted outdoors. To pre-vent the toxic effects, we now deploy home carbon monoxide monitors indoors to alert us of potentially hazardous CO exposure.

A second example of how outdoor concentrations and standards do not adequately reflect exposures and potential adverse health outcome is for the compound formaldehyde, a respiratory irritant and carcino-gen. While formaldehyde is emitted from outdoor combustion pro-cesses, including automobiles containing oxygenated fuels, and formed in the outdoor air by reactions of chemicals with sunlight, aldehydes can also be released from insulation used in homes. This can result in higher formaldehyde air concentrations indoors than outdoors [31].

The importance of indoor sources as a major contributor of air toxics to inhalation exposure is a lesson that still had not been learned as late as 2005–2006. In the aftermath of Hurricane Katrina, FEMA placed victims of the Hurricane in trailers that were laden with high levels of formaldehyde which resulted in many health-related complaints. This is a clear case of the need to understand total exposure and not just ambient air exposure to HAPs. Within the European Union, the Registration, Evaluation, Authorization and Restriction of Chemicals (REACH) program requires registration of all chemicals produced and imported into the European Union in quantities in excess of 1000 tons to assess their impact on both human health and the environment. Part of the chemical registration is the development of an exposure assessment that considers how products containing the chemical can lead to exposures through all exposure routes [32].

The box plots (Figure 1.2) for toluene and formaldehyde are based on data collected during the Relationship Among Indoor, Outdoor and Personal Air [33] study, and show that the mean and highest concentrations were observed in personal air, not outdoor air. A more detailed examination of the data show that for toluene, the personal exposure exceeded the residential indoor exposures, while for formaldehyde these two sample types were similar. This implies that for formaldehyde, residential indoor sources control inhalation exposure, while for toluene in addition to a strong residential source and outdoor contribution there are other sources leading to exposure. These include toluene exposures while driving, at service stations, and in places where smoking occurs. Thus, sources close to people and indoors can greatly increase the exposure above what is expected just from outdoor air.

1.3 EXPOSURE SCIENCE ACTIVITIES AND RISK ASSESSMENT

A formal use of modern exposure science began during the 1980s with the emergence of risk assessment as one of the tools to prioritize hazardous waste issues [34–36]. The completion of an exposure assessment was conceived as a simple data analysis tool to provide range "screening" results to determine the significance of the levels of toxicants at waste sites in terms of their "potential" to cause human health effects. It is one leg of the risk assessment equation that can provide a simple calculation of Risk = Exposure × Hazard. The actual determination of the exposure and hazard associated with an agent is highly dependent upon the type of health outcome, with cancer and noncancer endpoints having different averaging times in all cases, the exposure has to be measured or estimated to determine risk. There are many government documents available which prescribe step-by-step methods for using data and variables to estimate exposure and body burden. The goal usually is to have concentrations in units of mg/unit body weight-day. Thus, one can compare the contributions made by each route of entry into the body. The basic units for exposure and body burden used in these analyses are found in Table 1.1. The risk calculation has many assumptions which cause large uncertainties in estimating the risk for the presumed health effects. In particular, the assumptions used for a "screening" exposure estimate for the risk assessments at hazardous waste sites is not appropriate for exposure estimates made for other situations. At waste sites, the guidelines assumed contact by hypothetical individuals living and working on the

Table 1.1 Examples of Units Used to Express External and Internal Exposures

Variable	Typical Units	
Concentration in media	mg/kg	(food)
	mg/l or μg/l	(water)
	μg/m^3 and fibers/m^3	(air)
	mg/100 cm^2	(contaminated surface)
	mg/g or percent	(fraction by weight in consumer products)
Time increments	min, h, day, year, 70 years (lifetime)	
Rate of intake	l/day	
	l/h	
	mg/kg body weight ingested per day (or per meal)	
	mg inhaled per hour	
	Minutes	
Quantity available for absorption (potential dose)	mg inhaled, total	
	mg inhaled per kg body weight	
	mg ingested total	
	mg ingested per kg body weight	
	mg on skin, total	
	mg/cm^2 skin area	
	mg injected or implanted/kg body weight	
Concentration in body tissue	μg/ml blood fibers/ml lung tissue	
Body burden	μg in bone (example)	
Organ dose	mg to liver (example)	

un-remediated site for a lifetime to provide the maximum potential exposure rather than the actual exposure. While this might provide the maximum protection to the general public, it does not meet the practical needs in research or public health applications. Screening estimates have limited use in describing the types of remedial investigations needed to define the cleanup strategies, rather than represent a potential "realistic exposure."

An alternate approach was proposed within the Food Quality Protection Act (1996). It addressed total exposure by characterizing multiple compounds and aggregates multiple exposure routes [34]. The principles of exposure science required to estimate total exposure began to emerge in the 1990s, and are buttressed by the use of exposure information compiled by the USEPA and the implementation of similar requirements by a number of states.

Some of the initial concepts used to define exposure science can be found in the 1991 National Academy of Sciences report on *Human Exposure Assessment for Airborne Pollutants* where research needs were first identified and the tone for the future of the field set [35]. At the same time, a scientific journal was started, *Journal of Exposure Science* and *Environmental Epidemiology*. In addition, a scientific society, the International Society of Exposure Science (both formerly used the name Analysis for Science), was formed. Both continued to help define the field of exposure science [23,26,35,37].

REFERENCES

[1] Ramazzini B. Diseases of workers. New York, NY: Hafner Pub. Co.; 1964.

[2] Halliday S. The great stink of London, Sir Joseph Bazalgette and the cleansing of the victorian metropolis. Stroud, Gloucestershire: History Press, Sutton Publishing; 2009.

[3] Harris RL. The wheel of change. J Expo Anal Environ Epidemiol 1994;4:413−25.

[4] OSHA. <www.osha.gov/dsg/topics/pel>; 2013 [accessed October 2013].

[5] Inkret WC, Meinhold CB, Taschner JC. A brief history of radiation. Los Alamos Sci 1995;23:116−23.

[6] ICRP. P103: the 2007 recommendations of the international commission on radiological protection. ICRP 2007;37:1−332.

[7] ACGIH. TLVs and BEIs, Cincinnati, OH: 2013.

[8] US Congress. Clean Air Amendments of 1970. Public Law 91-604, 1970.

[9] Ott WR. Development of criteria for siting air monitoring stations. J Air Pollut Control Assoc 1977;27:543−7.

[10] US EPA. Air quality criteria for particulate matter. Washington, DC: U.S. Environmental Protection; 1969.

[11] NRC. Indoor pollutants. Washington, DC: The National Academies Press; 1981.

[12] Spengler J, Samet JM, McCarthy JF. Indoor air quality handbook. New York, NY: McGraw Hill; 2000.

[13] Smith KR. Total exposure assessment: part 1, implications for the U.S. Environment 1988;30:33−8 [10-5]

[14] Smith KR. Total exposure assesment: part 2, implications for developing countries. Environment 1988;30:16−20 8−35

[15] Wallace LA, Pellizzari ED, Hartwell TD, Sparacino CM, Sheldon L, Zelon H. Personal exposures, indoor−outdoor relationships, and breath levels of toxic air pollutants measured for 355 persons in New Jersey. Atmos Environ 1985;19:1651−61.

[16] Wallace LA, Pellizzari ED, Hartwell TD, Sparacino C, Whitmore R, Sheldon L, et al. The TEAM (Total Exposure Assessment Methodology) study: personal exposures to toxic substances in air, drinking water, and breath of 400 residents of New Jersey, North Carolina, and North Dakota. Environ Res 1987;43:290−307.

[17] Wallace LA. Major sources of benzene exposure. Environ Health Perspect 1989;82:165−9.

[18] Jo WK, Weisel CP, Lioy PJ. Routes of chloroform exposure and body burden from showering with chlorinated tap water. Risk Anal 1990;10:575−80.

[19] US EPA. Exposure factors handbook, EPA/600/P-95/002Fa,b,c. Washington, DC: U.S. Environmental Protection Agency; 1997.

[20] US EPA. Exposure factors handbook, EPA/600/R-09/052F. Washington, DC: U.S. Environmental Protection Agency; 2001.

[21] US EPA. Highlights of the exposure factors handbook, EPA/600/R-10/030. Washington, DC: U.S. Environmental Protection Agency; 2011.

[22] US EPA. Exposure factors handbook, EPA/600/R-09/052F. Washington, DC: U.S. Environmental Protection Agency; 2011.

[23] Lioy PJ. Assessing total human exposure to contaminants. A multidisciplinary approach. Environ Sci Tech 1990;24:938−45.

[24] Lioy PJ. Exposure science: a view of the past and milestones for the future. Environ Health Perspect 2010;118:1081−90.

[25] Ott W, Steinemann AC, Wallace LA. Exposure analysis. Boca Raton, FL: CRC Taylor & Francis; 2007.

[26] NRC. Exposure science in the 21st century: a vision and a strategy. Washington, DC: The National Academies Press; 2012.

[27] Ott WR. Human exposure assessment: the birth of a new science. J Expo Anal Environ Epidemiol 1995;5:449−72.

[28] US EPA. A conceptual framework for U.S. EPA's National Exposure Research Laboratory, EPA/000/R-09/003. Washington, DC: U.S. Environmental Protection Agency; 2009.

[29] Klaassen C. Casarett & Doull's toxicology: the basic science of poisons. 8th ed. New York, NY: McGraw Hill Professional; 2013.

[30] CDC. Third national report on human exposure to environmental chemicals executive summary. Atlanta, GA: Department of Health and Human Services, Centers for Disease Control and Prevention; 2005.

[31] Zhang J, Lioy PJ. Characteristics of aldehydes: concentrations, sources, and exposures for indoor and outdoor residential microenvironments. Environ Sci Technol 1994;28:146−52.

[32] The European Parliament and the Council of the European Union. 2006. Regulation (EC) No 1907/2006 of the European Parliament and of the Council of 18 December 2006: Official Journal of the European Union.

[33] Weisel CP, Zhang J, Turpin B, Morandi M, Colome S, Stock TH, et al. Relationship of Indoor, Outdoor and Personal Air (RIOPA) study: study design, methods and quality assurance/control results. J Expo Anal Environ Epidemiol 2005;123–37.

[34] NRC. Risk assessment in the federal government: managing the process. Washington, DC: The National Academies Press; 1983.

[35] NRC. Human exposure assessment for airborne pollutants:advances and opportunities. Washington, DC: The National Academies Press; 1991.

[36] NRC. Human biomonitoring for environmental chemicals. Washington, DC: The National Academies Press; 2006.

[37] Lioy PJ. The 1998 ISEA Wesolowski award lecture—exposure analysis: reflections on its growth and aspirations for its future. J Expo Anal Environ Epidemiol 1999;9:273–81.

CHAPTER 2

Definition of the Science and Mathematical Relationships

Today the field of exposure science as it relates specifically to humans is:

> The *"study of human contact with chemical, physical or biological agents occurring in their environments, and advanced knowledge of the mechanisms and dynamics of events either causing or preventing adverse health outcomes".*

This definition was published in the *Journal of Exposure Science and Environmental Epidemiology* in 2006 after a series of deliberations by a number of exposure scientists [1].

However, to understand the science's core principles, one must start with the definition of exposure which was first presented in the 1980s by Ott, Steinemann, and Wallace [2] as:

> *a person's contact with a material at a boundary (nose, skin or mouth) between the human and the "environment" at a concentration present in the environment over an interval of time.*

Today, based upon the evolution of the field and a recent NRC report, we need to augment this definition of exposure to:

> *A person's contact with the concentration of a material before and after it crosses a boundary (nose, skin or mouth) between the human and the environment over an interval of time leading to a potential biological effective dose* [3].

The reason for expanding the definition has been the recognition that biomarkers are an integral part of exposure science; this will become clear in subsequent sections and chapters, since it helps to establish coherence among the attributes that are ascribed to exposure.

In reaffirmation of a point made earlier, the key to the implementation of the principles of exposure science and its application within aligned fields of environmental health is a determination of whether or not a "contact" has occurred or can occur between the person and a toxic agent and the risk associated with that particular agent(s). A simple axiom to the above is that without any human contact or potential for human contact with a toxicant, there is no exposure and as a consequence no dose delivered to an organ or system. In the fifteenth century, Paracelsus stated that the "Dose makes the Poison" [4]. However for that term to be of utility to solving environmental and occupational health problems, Lioy augmented the statement as "exposure provides the dose that makes the poison" [5]. This is an important addition since it focuses attention on the bridge that exposure science provides between the presence of an agent in an environment and its ability to cause harm in a human. The contact or the plausibility of contact needs to be established before an exposure is definitively determined to have occurred and can cause harm, which is a challenge to investigators and many others.

Contacts and resulting exposure, however, can be either good or bad. For example, our ability to live each day starts with the continuous contact with and then an internal exposure to oxygen through breathing (inhalation exposure) which delivers a meaningful dose to and through the lungs for distribution to the circulatory system. In contrast, a short-term inhalation contact with chlorine or cyanide can lead to an exposure and then a biologically effective dose which can cause serious respiratory effects and, if the exposure level is high enough over a short period of time, death. These two examples also illustrate the major variables mentioned above, exposure time or duration, and concentration. Each of these variables is also tightly bound to the toxicity of a chemical or other agent. Together, exposure and toxicity indicate the plausibility of adverse health effects; thus, the emphasis on using biologically effective dose as the end point of an exposure to a toxic agent [6,7]. For a toxic agent of interest, the distribution and range of concentrations in an environment occupied by people needs to be established as does the time course or duration of any contacts that are meaningful in causing a health effect or positive (salutary) response associated with that agent. As a result, hypotheses can be generated about the dynamic processes that lead to contact and ultimately exposure. This is where environmental quality measurements differ from exposure measurements. The averaging time and duration of environmental sampling may be driven by measurement strategies associated with regulatory standards rather than where and how an individual contacts a toxic agent. The ability to quantify the exposure and then estimate or measure a meaningful dose is essential for defining a risk, e.g., what makes the poison. At this point in the discussion, we will introduce the mathematical equations used to describe exposure. In addition, a glossary of terminology commonly used in the field is also provided in Appendix A [8].

2.1 MATHEMATICAL REPRESENTATIONS OF EXPOSURE

Each of the routes of exposure is subject to study designs and model simulations that are controlled by the scientific principles and governing mathematical equations. The equations will be defined for total exposure or single route exposures. General external exposure Eqs. (2.1) and (2.2) are represented by [9,10].

$$E = \int_{t_0}^{t_1} C(t)\mathrm{d}t \tag{2.1}$$

and

$$E = \sum_{i=1}^{n} \Delta C_i \times \Delta t_i \quad i = 1 \text{ to } n \tag{2.2}$$

Equation (2.2) has been called the operational form of Eq. (2.1), because it is difficult to obtain continuous measurements within many environments and for each route of entry into the body. This is a reasonable statement since an infinite number of environments can be traversed by an individual over a period of time. Wayne Ott defined these discrete locations or situations as "microenvironments" [2]. The concept of microenvironment has been mostly applied to inhalation exposure to describe the locations people move in throughout the day and is continuous, since people continually breathe. Dermal contact and ingestion exposure are intermittent. Thus, such contacts can occur frequently or infrequently in a microenvironment or during activities over limited time periods.

Equation (2.1) represents the continuous integration of contact with a toxic agent for time varying concentrations, $C(t)$, from time t_0 to t_1, the interval or duration of contact. Equation (2.2) is the summation of the product of concentration and duration over n locations (microenvironments) or tasks (activities) that a person traverses over time. ΔC_i is the average concentration in each location or task, and Δt_i is the time spent in a location or completing a task (n). When using the equations, they are applied separately for each route of entry of an agent into the body. However, it is often necessary to understand all routes of exposure, i.e., total exposure, to establish meaningful exposure–health outcome relationship.

Since Eq. (2.1) requires knowledge of the continuous exposure for the entire time period, it is rarely used to examine a problem. However, new real-time sensors and methods to continuously log activities may make the application of this equation more practical in the future, particularly for inhalation routes.

Equation (2.2), which is more commonly used to characterize exposure in various settings, is the summation of all or most of the "contacts" that lead to exposures. Locations can be the home, outdoors in a city, or the office.

The evolution of the field over the past 30 years has led to the following mathematical constructs. These were first published by Duan, and later modified by Georgopoulos and Lioy [11,15]. If modified slightly, Eq. (2.1) provides a means of describing exposure for all possible cases over time for a given route of entry into the body. For all routes of entry into the body, Eqs. (2.1) and (2.2) actually are the representations of external exposure, or the levels which approach a boundary or surface over time and are associated with a route of entry into the body. However, since the units associated with contact at each boundary are not the same, we cannot readily combine routes of exposure together (see Table 1.1) Thus, a new equation, Eq. (2.3), is presented to describe an individual exposure route, r, (inhalation, ingestion, dermal, etc.) one at a time. The external exposure concentration for route, r, is integrated over time to calculate exposure $E_{ext,r}$ (concentration $\times$ time) Eq. (2.3):

$$E_{ext,r} = \int_0^t C_r \, dt \qquad (2.3)$$

where r is one of the four routes of exposure.

For a single route of exposure and multiple (j) discontinuous exposure events over an exposure period the form of the Eq. (2.4) is:

$$E_t = \sum_1^j \int_0^t C_r \, dt \qquad (2.4)$$

This is analogous to Eq. (2.2), except it is a summation of discrete intervals of integrated exposure rather than average exposures multiplied by duration.

For a human exposure associated with route r, a high C, and a short t would be associated with acute affects, while a lower concentration of (C) over longer times would be meaningful for chronic or long-term health outcomes. Thus, as stated above, knowledge of biological half times is a prerequisite for establishing a defensible exposure (E) for a particular impact (Figure 2.1) [13]. Being unable to directly sum over all r routes of entry into the body is a general problem in using external exposure as the main metric within the field.

The incompatibility mentioned above was an issue for Eqs. (2.1)–(2.4). Lioy identified this problem and proposed using internal dose (D_{in}) as a solution to this mathematical discontinuity since the contributions of external exposures across routes of entry into the body could be expressed with a common unit, an amount present in the body over an interval of time [14]. This concept was considered within the most recent NRC committee on exposure [3]. That committee's deliberations resulted in an important new term for exposure science: Internal exposure (E_{int}) which is equivalent to D_{in}. E_{int} is a

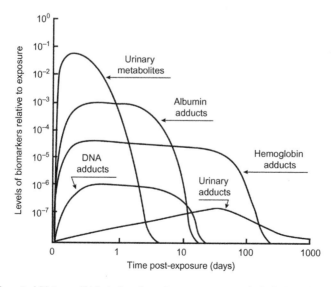

Figure 2.1 Theoretical lifetimes of biological markers of exposure present in the body. Reproduced with permission from Ref. [13].

function of all routes of entry, r, and can be represented mathematically as Eq. (2.5):

$$E_{int} = \int f(x_j, t)g(ab)C(t))P(e)dt \qquad (2.5)$$

where $f(x_j, t)$ is the contact rate over time, $g(ab)$ is the fraction absorbed including bioavailability and is dependent upon the boundary layer, $P(e)$ is the fraction eliminated from a fluid or tissue.

The NRC determined that to properly understand and quantify exposure, the amount of a toxicant present within the body is just as important as the exposure estimated or measured at the external contact points for each route of entry into the body. Since internal exposure can be expressed in the same units as other relevant measures and estimates made by other applications (e.g., toxicology, epidemiology, and risk assessment), internal exposure permits direct comparisons of data interpreted across disciplines.

Internal exposure (E_{int}) has been defined in the NRC report as:

Contact between an agent and a human one level of physical or biological organization past the external boundary towards the site of action for the agent (e.g. a tissue, cell or molecular receptor) [3].

It describes the measurements made beyond the traditional external boundaries defined by Ott, Steinemann, and Wallace [2] and can include quantitative concentration data for various bodily fluids and tissues, e.g., blood or urine.

The calculation of internal exposure provides a unit of the mass of an agent that has crossed an absorption boundary at a contact surface. It requires representing the process directly as a rate of transport or indirectly as a composite term representing the net fraction of material reaching the contact surface which becomes the internalized mass reaching a body tissue, e.g., blood. This is calculated based on f, the bioavailability for the specific boundary, system or organ, and V, the volume of the media that absorbs or adsorbs the agent (Eq. (2.6)):

$$E_{int} = f \times \int_0^t C(t) x \frac{V}{t} dt \qquad (2.6)$$

The E_{int} can be eventually become part of modeling equations, including physiologically based pharmacokinetic (PBPK) information, needed to calculate a biologically relevant or effective dose. Based upon Eq. (2.6), two modifications are required to calculate concentrations (mass/volume) at the receptor location of interest. The addition of one or more terms to describe removal or elimination of the material from the receptor (k_{elim}, mass/time), and the volume of the receptor (volume of distribution, VD, 1/volume) Eq. (2.7):

$$E_{\text{int,r}} = f \times \frac{1}{\text{VD}} \int_0^t C(t)x\frac{V}{t}\,dt - k_{\text{elim}}\,dt \tag{2.7}$$

for $r = 1$ to 4.

Conveniently, this form of the equation is consistent with those used extensively in the toxicology, medical and pharmaceutical industries to describe the pharmacokinetics of drugs and chemicals. The terms included describe adsorption (f), distribution (VD), and metabolism/elimination (k_{elim}). More complete pharmacokinetic/mass transport equations can be substituted for each of these terms to be more physiology representative, ultimately these revised variables lead to models of internal exposure which are known as PBPK and physiologically based toxicokinetic (PBTK) models [15].

To summarize, the preceding concepts are consistent with those published by Lioy and recently discussed by Cohen-Hubel [6,14]. Redefining Eq. (2.3) as an internal exposure, E_{int}, allows the measurements made for biological markers of exposure in, for example, blood and urine, to be properly interpreted within exposure science, as a convenient end point for estimating internal exposure from external marker data that include behavior and activity patterns. It can provide a quantitative basis for comparing the relative importance of each route of exposure, and when combined with a toxicological understanding, their importance in addressing a health impact.

The internal exposure across multiple routes of exposure can be calculated using Eq. (2.8):

$$E_{\text{totalint}} = \frac{1}{\text{VD}}\left(\left(\sum_1^x f_r x \int_0^t C(t)x\frac{V}{t}\,dt\right) - k_{\text{elim}}\,dt\right) \tag{2.8}$$

Using this equation, the levels of exposure for each route (r) can actually be estimated or calculated and the most significant route of entry prioritized in a mathematically consistent form. Finally, the concept of internal exposure can be further extended using PBTK modeling. The latter has been available for many years to address the importance of measuring and quantifying the dose at the site of action at a specific tissue, cell or protein receptor in an organism, or within a specific compartment of an ecosystem.

The use of the term "internal exposure" can be easily used in both conceptual and theoretical discussions, and experimental design [6]. The quantitative definition of internal exposure is the same as the term internal dose discussed by Lioy, but is now embraced as part of exposure science as examined by the NRC [3,14,15]. Internal exposure values can be used to establish quantitative coherency in the units used to describe the exposure values associated with different routes of entry into a human as well as related fields of toxicology, risk assessment, risk management, and clinical medicine.

2.2 A UNIFIED APPROACH TO THE SOURCE TO IMPACT CONTINUUM

With the extension and refinement of the term exposure to comprise two more specific concepts: external and internal, the field now has a language and mathematical term that directly correlates with terms used in the medical, pharmaceutical, and toxicological fields, e.g., administered dose, intake/uptake dose, and biologically effective dose. These and the associated concepts and equations for quantifying exposure form a modified conceptual framework for the field (Figure 2.2). Thus, hypotheses can be generated around questions related to either internal or external exposures. The application of the conceptual framework for the source to impact continuum outlined in Figure 2.2 will not always be directed or preferentially directed toward the center, the impact. In fact, to be truly of value to the large range of applications, the analyses could also be bidirectional, i.e., toward or away from the center (toward the source), or just directed away from the center [3,16]. Exposure applications for epidemiology, risk assessment, and intervention can primarily be directed toward the center. Conversely, the applications related to prevention, engineering or administrative control, and policy can be directed away from the center and toward activities aligned with exposure science, e.g., regulations, standards, and product or process replacement.

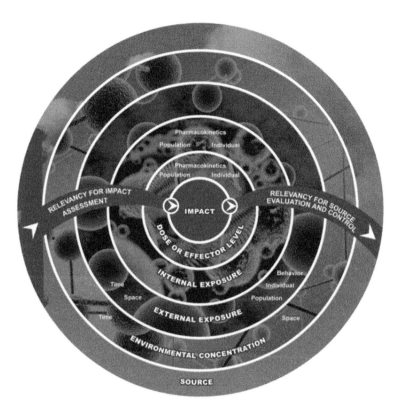

Figure 2.2 Exposure science as applied at any level of biologic organization from the external environment to the dose at a target site. Reproduced with permission from Ref. [3].

Exposure science can be applied at any level of biological organization: The ecological level, community level, or individual level, and within the individual level, at the level of external exposure, internal exposure, or target site exposure [3]. The uncertainties in applications of exposure science for each of the preceding will still be dependent upon whether the external exposure provides a meaningful representation of the exposure–response relationship. Thus, in some cases, using environmental monitoring data as an estimate of exposure will still be sufficient if the user is provided with data such as activity patterns and the duration of exposure. In other cases, use of internal exposure measures would be more logical, e.g., when examining exposure–response relationships among children with a lead burden.

For the inverse process, any one of many different metrics of exposure can be useful in helping define the source in Figure 2.2 and reduce uncertainty. Thus, the value of exposure metrics in the control and prevention of exposure derived from one or more sources clearly is an important and significant component in the implementation of the framework.

REFERENCES

[1] Barr DB. Human exposure science: a field of growing importance. J Expo Sci Environ Epidemiol 2006;16:473.

[2] Ott W, Steinemann AC, Wallace LA. Exposure analysis. Boca Raton, FL: CRC Taylor & Francis; 2007.

[3] NRC. Exposure science in the 21st century: a vision and a strategy. Washington, DC: The National Academies Press; 2012.

[4] Klaassen C. Casarett & Doull's toxicology: the basic science of poisons. 8th ed. New York, NY: McGraw Hill Professional; 2013.

[5] Lioy PJ. Exposure science: a view of the past and milestones for the future. Environ Health Perspect 2010;118:1081−90.

[6] Cohen-Hubal EA. Biologically relevant exposure science for 21st century toxicity testing. Toxicol Sci 2009;111:226−32.

[7] Lioy PJ. Exposure analysis and the biological response to a contaminant: a melding necessary for environmental health science. J Expo Anal Environ Epidemiol 1992;Suppl. 1:1−244.

[8] Zartarian V, Bahadori T, McKone TE. Adoption of an offical ISEA glossary. J Expo Anal Environ Epidemiol 2005;15:1−5.

[9] NRC. Human exposure assessment for airborne pollutants: advances and opportunities. Washington, DC: The National Academies Press; 1991.

[10] Duan N. Models for human exposure to air pollution. Environ Int 1982;8:305−9.

[11] Duan N. Stochastic microenvironment models for air pollution exposure. J Expo Anal Environ Epidemiol 1991;1:235−57.

[12] Lioy PJ, Smith KR. A discussion of exposure science in the 21st century: a vision and a strategy. Environ Health Perspect 2013;121:405−9.

[13] Henderson R, Bechtold WE, Bond JA, Sun JD. The use of biological markers in toxicology. Crit Rev Toxicol 1989;20:65−82.

[14] Lioy PJ. Assessing total human exposure to contaminants. A multidisciplinary approach. Environ Sci Technol 1990;24:938−45.

[15] Georgopoulos PG, Lioy PJ. From a theoretical framework of human exposure and dose assessment to computational system implementation: the Modeling Environment for Total Risk Studies (MENTOR). J Toxicol Environ Health 2006;9:457−83.

[16] Georgopoulos PG, Sasso AF, Isukapalli SS, Lioy PJ, Vallero DA, Okino M, et al. Reconstructing population exposures to environmental chemicals from biomarkers: challenges and opportunities. J Environ Sci Technol 2009;19:149−71.

CHAPTER 3

Exposure Routes and Types of Exposure

The simple application of Eq. (2.2) to calculate external exposure by multiplying the average concentration in that location by how long a time the person (s) spent there or $E = C \times t$ can provide erroneous predictions about possible adverse health effects. Even this simple calculation requires the use of significant judgment with respect to a health outcome. For example, assume that for acute toxicant A, contact time of 2 h at a minimum concentration of 100 parts per billion is needed to cause an adverse health effect. Multiplying these values together yields an exposure value of 200 ppb-h. This implies that an exposure to an acute toxicant at or above this value would yield a meaningful exposure. However, without knowledge of the time and concentration relationship for the specific health effect, the total value of E could be meaningless. An exposure value of 200 ppb-h can be the result of an infinite number of combinations of concentration and time. For instance a 20 h exposure at 10 ppb would yield a value of 200 but would have little to no effect on the health of an individual or population for this specific toxicant which only exerts an acute effect at higher concentrations. Thus, except for limited circumstances, this simple multiplication does not work, and more complex mathematical representations of exposure are needed.

As mentioned above, two exposure concepts associated with all routes of exposure are [1]:

1. *Contact rate*: The rate at which an agent reaches a boundary and then crosses it and enters the body. To be of most value for interpretation of exposure for risk assessment and comparisons across different routes of entry into the body, the units should be a volume or surface area over unit time or event. Typically, for inhalation amount per m^3, for liquid ingestion amount per liter, for food amount per kg, and for dermal amount per cm^2 of surface per unit time (hour or day). As shown in the preceding equations (2.5, 2.6), these values are essential for estimating the internal exposure or back calculating external exposure.

2. *Total exposure*: The total amount of a material received by a person from all sources and microenvironments over the time of interest. Total exposure would be derived from all routes of entry into the body. This concept has at times been used to explain exposure for a single route.

For the purposes of this book, internal and external exposure is differentiated from the dose at a target organ that leads to a health outcome, which we have specifically identified as a biological effective dose. A biologically effect dose has been defined as:

the quantity (concentration) of a substance that produces harmful or healthy biological response(s) at one or more sites of action.

Toxicologists call internal exposure, the internal or administered dose. As stated previously, internal exposure provides a metric for comparisons of the level and intensity of exposures across all routes of entry into the body (ingestion, inhalation, dermal, and injection). By estimating or measuring internal exposure, it is possible to have a reasonable metric for comparing exposures extrapolated from models or measurements to health based standards based upon body burdens.

The mathematical concepts for estimating internal exposure provides a basis for cross disciplinary analyses. We will use risk assessment to demonstrate that coherence. The equations for external and internal exposure are not new. The discrete version of the $E_{int,r}$ (combination of Eqs. (2.2) and (2.7)) is Eq. (3.1)):

$$\Delta E_{int,r} = f \times \frac{1}{VD} \Delta C \frac{xV}{t} - K_{elim} \Delta t \qquad (3.1)$$

has been employed since the 1980s to characterize exposure assessment for risk assessment. The calculation used in an exposure assessment for risk assessment usually refers to the internal exposure as *an intake or absorbed dose*. The basic mathematical formulations are found in various EPA superfund guidance documents (see example below) [2]. The logic was simple: the risk associated with each exposure route needed to be prioritized. To make a comparison across the routes, the exposures needed to be expressed in equivalent units and be related to health based standards. Intake was usually expressed as mg/kg-day. The calculations are straightforward and use the typical exposure factors and environmental concentration values to calculate the internal exposure (intake or absorbed dose). As an example, the mathematical formulation for contaminant intake from water ingestion is as follows Eq. (3.2):

$$\text{Intake (agent } \times) = C \text{ (mg/}l) \times \text{IR } (l/\text{day}) \times \text{EF (days/year)} \times \text{ED (exposure duration)}/\text{BW (kg)} \times \text{AT (day)} \tag{3.2}$$

where C is the concentration of an agent, IR (contact rate) is the ingestion rate, EF is the exposure frequency, ED is the exposure duration, BW is the body weight, and AT is the averaging time. Similar equations exist for the inhalation and dermal routes of entry into the body.

Total internal exposure can be estimated using appropriate biological marker measurements. However, biomarkers usually do not differentiate the amount that comes from each route of entry into the body. That knowledge requires external markers of exposure and the associated behaviors and activities.

3.1 TOTAL EXPOSURE

Total exposure as defined above for a person or population is the "exposures across all routes over a period of time." The duration can be short, <1 h to very long, $\gg$ year. Total exposure characterization is often not a straightforward process since it incorporates many variables, including human activities and behavior which can be difficult to characterize. In addition, the contacts and resulting exposures can be discrete, repetitive, or continuous, and involve many microenvironments and activities. However, total exposure can be estimated when the number of covariables is reduced [1].

Estimating total exposure from the equations for internal exposure is difficult since the factors needed are not routinely available over appropriate time intervals. For example, Eq. (2.5) requires at a minimum the bioavailability or bioaccessibility and the elimination rate of the target agent to calculate an internal exposure in the various bodily fluids and tissues impacted. An alternate approach to estimate internal exposure is to use Eq. (3.2) for risk assessment. That would focus on estimates of contact rates, $f(x)$, followed by a determination of accumulation in the affected bodily fluids, etc.

3.1.1 Approaches to Exposure Characterizations

The general approaches to characterize exposure are measurements, model estimates, or a combination of both. Currently, except for some occupational situations or specific environmental cases [3−10], there usually are too few measurements and too little information on human activities available to completely model the exposure. Even the mean, and high (~95‰) and low exposures (~5‰) need to be estimated in many environmental situations [11−13]. The measurement approach should ideally include a field study that relies heavily on personal monitoring combined with documentation of activities to establish the plausibility that "contact" occurs and to potentially identify the sources of the agent(s) of concern. In the absence of personal sampling, exposure modeling can be used to fill large gaps in information with varying levels of uncertainty about exposure concentrations and activities using extant databases. Regulatory situations that involve exposure based standards, not just environmental quality, many times use extant databases containing concentrations in different media and human activity patterns to prospectively estimate high or consequential exposures [13]. These models, as will be explained later in the book, are not just environmental fate and transport models, but rather human exposure models [12,14−24]. The former describes the toxicant's movement in the environment and the latter describes human contact with the toxicant. For either case, the application of exposure science to environmental or occupational health problems can be considered a "receptor oriented approach." This has been expressed in the literature by Ott et al. and is a reasonable way to focus on the impact of the field in evaluating the causes of exposure and ways for reducing or eliminating those causes of exposure [1]. It is opposite of the approach usually taken by regulatory agencies. They traditionally focus on the sources and then the impact on a local or larger population. Before the creation of environmental and occupational regulatory agencies in the United States, Europe, and elsewhere, ambient pollution routinely occurred at levels that adversely affected public health, via acute or chronic exposures. Thus, it was relatively easy to focus attentions on source control rather than receptor impacts, e.g., London smog [25]. As emissions from many industrial and transportation sources have been reduced in developed countries, the resulting levels of air and water pollution from those "traditional" sources have become less important as the dominant pathway for exposure routes of entry into the body. Relatively smaller pollutant releases close to an individual or discrete population are becoming more important. However, the high exposure situations from industrial and transportation sources for both acute and chronic air and waterborne exposures persist in many developing countries.

One example of the move from exposures related to traditional sources to those related to less apparent sources is lead. In many countries, after the ban on lead in gasoline went into effect, the significance of direct lead emissions from cars on inhalation was reduced to deminimus levels [26–28]. However, there is still a legacy of health effects from lead exposure derived from soil, street dust, flaking paint, etc. Thus, an inhalation exposure issue has been reorientated to become an incidental ingestion issue. There are still sources of lead in the United States that result in inhalation exposure, i.e., resuspended dust. However, in other parts of the world where lead is still added to gasoline as an antiknock agent, inhalation exposure still dominates the total exposure to lead. This straightforward example illustrates the process used to triage routes of exposure during the analysis of total exposure. For other agents, the process of characterizing total exposure or prioritizing the importance of individual routes of exposure may be more complex. This is now being recognized for chemicals in consumer products and pesticides used in homes.

3.2 CUMULATIVE AND AGGREGATE EXPOSURES

To deal with the issue of prioritization by route or multiple agents, in the mid-1990s, the concepts of cumulative and aggregate exposures were introduced to provide a basic framework to address total exposure issues using measurement and monitoring strategies. They are defined as follows:

Cumulative exposure is the contact/exposure of an individual or defined population to multiple agents with the same toxic effects found in at least one environmental medium and released by one or more sources [29].

Aggregate exposure is the contact or exposure of a defined population or individual to a single agent from all relevant sources and all relevant routes of entry into the body [30].

Measurement or modeling research designs for cumulative exposure focus primarily on multiple agents across one route of exposure (e.g., diet). The agents selected should have similar health endpoints (e.g., neurological) and be present in one environmental medium. A general mixture associated with one or more sources that contribute to that route of exposure route can also be considered cumulative. In contrast, aggregate exposure provides a much more targeted or focused approach for measurements and analyses. It is used to evaluate the contributions from one or more exposure routes to an individual or populations for a single toxic agent. In the 1990s, these concepts were the basis of a major research design used to examine pesticide exposures to achieve the goals of the Food Quality Protection Act (FQPA) [31].

Box 3.1 provides an example of aggregate exposure. Contaminants in drinking water could be thought of as a problem due to consumption of water. However, a detailed exposure analysis reveals that there are multiple routes that contribute to the total exposure, as illustrated for chloroform, a disinfection by-product of chlorine added to drinking water.

Exposures routes are the actual portals of entry for a toxicant into the human body. They were described mathematically for each route, r, for both external and internal exposures in Eqs. (2.3) and (2.7), respectively. As shown in the continuum Figure 1.1, once the toxicant has entered the body, the focus of attention eventually turns from internal exposure to biologically effective dose. The levels of interaction between the release of a toxic agent in an exposure pathway and the individual or population [3,16,17] depend upon the significance of individual routes of exposure.

3.3 THE FOUR ROUTES OF EXPOSURE

Inhalation: This involves breathing a toxicant resulting in direct contact at one or more of the three major regions of the respiratory system: nasal-pharynx (nose, mouth, and pharynx), the thoracic (the bronchial tree), and air exchange region (bronchioles and the alveoli sacs) (Figure 3.1).

Each of these regions can be affected by an exposure to a chemical (e.g., benzene, carbon monoxide), physical (e.g., nuclear radiation), or biological agent (e.g., virus, bacteria, or mold). Deposition or absorption of species occurs differently in each region based on the solubility

---

Box 3.1 Aggregate Exposure to Chloroform in Tap Water, a By-Product of Chlorination

The obvious route of chloroform exposure is ingestion since tap water is drunk and used in food preparation. The amounts and frequency of drinking beverages (including water itself) or foods prepared with tap water through the time period of interest, often 24 h, need to be determined along with the water concentration in each beverage and food. The latter can vary since chloroform concentration can change throughout the day as it is delivered to a faucet. If the water is filtered at the tap or in the home, the chloroform will be reduced or in unfiltered situations, it can evaporate from an open beverage or heated food. People consume beverages and food at various locations throughout the day (home, office, school, restaurant), each having potentially different chloroform water concentration. Water is used multiple ways besides being ingested that can lead to alternate exposure routes. Water is used for washing, showering, bathing, laundry, cleaning, swimming, etc. For inhalation exposure, the release of chloroform from the water into different locations can travel within a number of microenvironments where people spend time. For example, breathing air within a shower stall has been identified contributing to more than 20% of the total chloroform daily exposure [24]. In addition, the chloroform released during showering, washing dishes, running washing machine, and dishwashers contribute to the indoor chloroform air concentration resulting in inhalation exposure to all members of a household [32]. Showering and bathing result in dermal exposures to chloroform as do swimming and washing dishes [33]. Obtaining the data necessary to determine exposure can be a composite of measurement, observations, surveys, and mathematical modeling. However, the units of external exposure are the same (concentration in air per day, amount contacting the skin per day, amount ingested per day), so summation across routes is not possible in the form presented by Eq. (2.1) Use Eq. (3.2).

---

for gaseous species in the respiratory lining fluid or the size and shape for particulate species [34]. In the extra-thoracic region, highly soluble gaseous species are absorbed and super coarse, large particles are deposited ($>10\,\mu m$) [35]. In the tracheobronchial region, the airways go through a series of dichotomous branching which result in an increasing linear velocity of the breath and deposition of smaller particles. The bronchiole is the gas-exchange region of the respiratory tract and the final location for particles to deposit until the breath is expired by an individual. The location where particles deposit in the respiratory tract, the extent of solubilization of different particles, and their

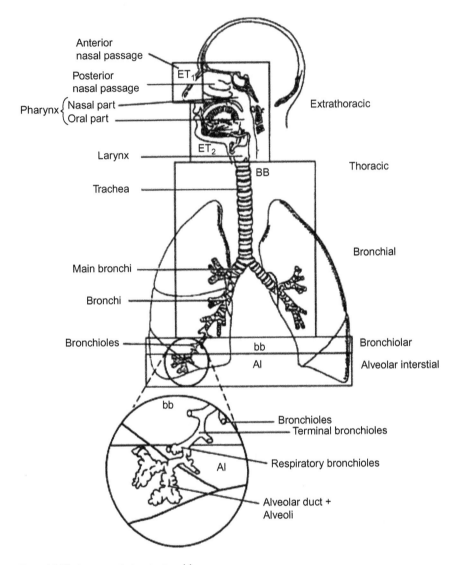

Figure 3.1 The human respiratory tract model.

interaction with or absorption through the respiratory lining contribute to their bioavailability (Eq. (2.5)). These affect the internal exposure and are important considerations in any adverse health outcome of exposure, e.g., respiratory disease.

The internal exposure from inhalation is a function of not only the air concentration of the agent being breathed but also the breathing rate (contact) of the individual. An individual who is exercising or involved in manual labor will breathe faster and more deeply than someone at rest resulting in their receiving a higher exposure delivered further into the respiratory tract from the same air concentration. Air concentrations contacting a person vary spatially and temporally as he or she moves. The air concentration being breathed at any point in time is dependent upon the person's proximity to sources, whether the emissions are occurring within an enclosed microenvironment or in an open space, and the presence of ventilation. In addition, whether or not the exposure is acute (peak) and/or chronic (average over time) impacts the health identifiers of endpoint of concern. Inhalation exposure can be directly linked to the site of injury in the respiratory tract. For other adverse health outcomes, the internal exposure from inhalation can be quantified using the air concentration and characterization of the toxicants (e.g., constituents on particles), duration of contact, breathing rate, and uptake across the lung boundary.

Ingestion: This involves the consumption either intentionally (dietary) or inadvertently (nondietary) of nutrients (beneficial) and toxicants (harmful). Contaminated food or beverages are the most obvious sources of ingestion of a toxicant. Chemical or biological contamination of food can occur during the production, processing, transportation, preparation/cooking, serving, or eating of food. Examples are the uptake of a toxicant from contaminated soil, the presence of toxicants in animal feed, the spraying of pesticides onto a food surface, and the transference of contaminants to food from surfaces during preparation or handling in homes (e.g., dragging a lollipop on a rug). Similarly, in a food processing facility, *E. coli* contamination is caused by improper hygienic practices by workers, or improper storage or transport of food. Intentional adulteration of food can also occur through the use of inappropriate fillers for economic reasons or by individuals seeking to cause harm to an individual or population. Contaminated drinking water can be consumed directly or used in food or beverage preparation. Chemical contaminants include metals and organic compounds. Organic contaminants concentrations can bioaccumulate/biomagnify (increase) in the tissue of edible species as one moves up the food chain. Identifying populations or individuals that have been or likely to be exposed to contaminated food or drinking water requires an understanding of activity and behavior patterns of individuals, including cultural considerations, to understand what and how often foods are likely to be eaten and how one prepares the food.

Incidental or inadvertent ingestion occurs when a person, particularly a child, ingests contaminated soil or house dust, or chews or sucks on contaminated objects [36,37]. A better term is simply nonfood ingestion since the amount and frequency may not be incidental. Chewing or sucking objects (including contaminated hands and fingers) are a common exposure pathway for pesticide and lead exposures. Nonfood ingestion exposure can occur in adults when individuals place items such as cigarettes that had touched contaminated surfaces, in their mouth, a situation noted to occur in occupational settings. Hand-to-mouth contact frequency in children studied using videotaping are ~ 10 and ~ 20 contacts/h for 2–6 and 0.5–2 year olds, respectively [38]. These activities have often been underreported in simple questionnaires completed by parents and caretakers, which highlights the need for rigorous methodologies to determine human activities [39–41].

Over the past 15 years, the scientific community has become more aware that surface dust can be a reservoir for lead, pesticides, and semivolatile species released and redistributed indoors [42,43]. Transference of dust contaminants onto food from hands that are not washed before eating, or if hands directly touch the mouth, results in food and nonfood ingestion exposure pathways for both children and adults.

Ingestion exposure from food is calculated from the contaminant level in food and the quantity consumed. Tracing the contamination of food through the entire food system can be difficult due to the large variety of food consumed, each with many potential sources of contamination. Determination of types and quantity of food consumed requires detailed evaluation of the activity of individual(s). As part of this evaluation, information on when and if a transference/formation of contaminants occurred within the home or during food preparation/cooking can be examined. Nondietary exposure estimates can be made from measurements of levels on hands or biomarker levels. Biomarker levels reflect internal exposures across all routes as modified by compound metabolism and excretion from the body. For ingestion exposure, the net amount of an agent that is absorbed from the digestive system, i.e., the internal exposure, needs to consider the bioaccessibility/bioavailability of the agent from the food, soil, or dust ingested by a person rather than just the total amount consumed by an individual [44,45].

Dermal: This involves the contact between the skin and a toxicant on surfaces or in the air. Toxicants associated with dermal exposure can cause skin irritation or be absorbed into the body (e.g., chloroform during showering or bathing) through the epidermis (Figure 3.2). Intact skin epidermis provides a protective barrier to many agents (bacteria, metal ions) but is permeable to lipophilic compounds. The hands are the most prominent portion of the body that contacts the surroundings directly, outside of showering, bathing, or swimming. Clothing protects other portions of the body to a limited extent. However, if clothing becomes wet, it can facilitate the dermal exposure by being a repository for agents which can then be transported through the epidermis. Clothing may also not be an effective barrier for vapors [46,47]. Penetration through the skin can vary across different parts of the body due to differences in the thickness of the epidermis. The lipophilic nature of a contaminant is a primary determinant for the amount of penetration of a compound through the skin. Within the occupational settings, personal protection is often worn to avoid dermal absorption, but the degree of protection is dependent upon the materials used in the protective gear and the agents or carriers that the protective gear is designed to interdict the contact and exposure. Additionally, at times individuals might forego the use of protective equipment because it is too hot and uncomfortable; there is a lack of access to equipment because of economics; because individuals are unaware of the need due

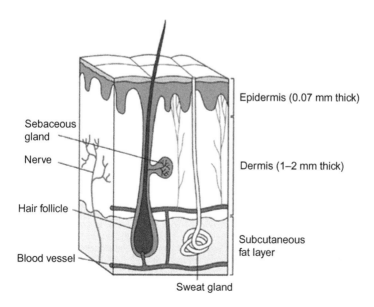

Figure 3.2 The layers of the human skin that can be affected by dermal exposure.

to lack of training; or because the protective equipment use precludes completing a job in a timely manner. Dermal absorption of vapors from volatile or semivolatile agents can also occur but is typically smaller than from liquids contacting the skin [46,47].

Injection: This is the penetration of a toxicant into the body via an external agent such as during vaccination, sex, or other activity, legal or illegal. Occasionally penetration can also occur from particles or materials that are emitted at high speed and contact the skin. This can cause material to be embedded within the skin that can lead to a rash or continued systemic release of agents [48].

REFERENCES

[1] Ott W, Steinemann AC, Wallace LA. Exposure analysis. Boca Raton, FL: CRC Taylor & Francis; 2007.

[2] US EPA. Guidelines for exposure assessment, EPA/600/Z-92/001. Washington, DC: U.S Environmental Protection, Risk Assessment Forum; 1992.

[3] Georgopoulos PG, Sasso AF, Isukapalli SS, Lioy PJ, Vallero DA, Okino M, et al. Reconstructing population exposures to environmental chemicals from biomarkers: challenges and opportunities. J Environ Sci Technol 2009;19:149−71.

[4] Clayton CA, Perritt RL, Pellizzari ED, Thomas KW, Whitmore RW, Wallace LA, et al. Particle Total Exposure Assessment Methodology (PTEAM) study: distributions of aerosol and elemental concentrations in personal, indoor, and outdoor air samples in a Southern California community. J Expo Anal Environ Epidemiol 1993;3:227−50.

[5] Freeman NC, Stern AH, Lioy PJ. Exposure to chromium dust from homes in a chromium surveillance project. Arch Environ Health 1997;52:213−9.

[6] Heinrich J, Holscher B, Seiwert M, Carty CL, Merkel G, Schulz C. Nicotine and cotinine in adults' urine: The German Environmental Survey 1998. J Expo Anal Environ Epidemiol 2005;15:74−80.

[7] Hoffmann K, Krause C, Seifert B, Ullrich D. The German Environmental Survey 1990/92 (GerES II): sources of personal exposure to volatile organic compounds. J Expo Anal Environ Epidemiol 2000;10:115−25.

[8] Jantunen MJ, Hanninen O, Katsouyanni K, Knoppel H, Kuenzli N, Lebret E, et al. Air pollution exposure in European cities: the "EXPOLIS" study. J Expo Anal Environ Epidemiol 1998;8:495−518.

[9] Pellizzari E, Lioy PJ, Quackenboss J, Whitmore R, Clayton A, Freeman N, et al. Population-based exposure measurements in EPA region 5: a phase I field study in support of the National Human Exposure Assessment Survey. J Expo Anal Environ Epidemiol 1995;5:583.

[10] Schreiber JS. An exposure and risk assessment regarding the presence of tetrachlorethene in human breast milk. J Expo Anal Environ Epidemiol 1992;2:15−26.

[11] Lebowitz M, Lioy PJ, McKone TE, Spengler J, Adgate JL, Bennett D, et al. The necessity of observing children's exposure of contaminants in their real-world environmental settings; 2008.

[12] Lebowitz MD, Quackenboss JJ, Kollander M, Soczek ML, Colome S. The new standard environmental inventory questionnaire for estimation of indoor concentrations. J Air Pollut Control Assoc 1989;39:1411–9.

[13] US EPA. EPA's Stochastic Human Exposure and Dose Simulation (SHEDS) model. Washington, DC: U.S Environmental Protection Agency; 2012.

[14] Duan N. Models for human exposure to air pollution. Environ Int 1982;8:305–9.

[15] Duan N. Stochastic microenvironment models for air pollution exposure. J Expo Anal Environ Epidemiol 1991;1:235–57.

[16] Lioy PJ, Smith KR. A discussion of exposure science in the 21st century: a vision and a strategy. Environ Health Perspect 2013;121:405–9.

[17] Georgopoulos PG, Wang SW, Georgopoulos IG, Yonone-Lioy MJ, Lioy PJ. Assessment of human exposure to copper: a case study using the NHEXAS database. J Expo Sci Environ Epidemiol 2006;16:397–409.

[18] Glen G, Smith L, Isaacs K, McCurdy T, Langstaff J. A new method of longitudinal diary assembly for human exposure modeling. J Expo Sci Environ Epidemiol 2008;18:299–311.

[19] Jerrett M, Arain A, Kanaroglou P, Beckerman B, Potoglou D, Sahsuvaroglu T, et al. A review and evaluation of intraurban air pollution exposure models. J Expo Anal Environ Epidemiol 2005;15:185–204.

[20] Johnson T, Capel J. A Monte Carlo approach to simulating residential occupancy periods and its application to the general U.S. population. Research Triangle Park, NC: U.S. Environmental Protection Agency; 1992.

[21] McCurdy T, Glen G, Smith L, Lakkadi Y. The national exposure research laboratory's consolidated human activity database. J Expo Anal Environ Epidemiol 2000;10:566–78.

[22] Mckone TE. Human exposure to chemicals from multiple media and through multiple pathways—research overview and comments. Risk Anal 1991;11:5–10.

[23] NRC. Models in environmental regulatory decision making. Washington, DC: The National Academies Press; 2007.

[24] Price PS, Chaisson CF. A conceptual framework for modeling aggregate and cumulative exposures to chemicals. J Expo Anal Environ Epidemiol 2005;15:473–81.

[25] Vallero D. Fundamentals of air pollution. 4th ed. Burlington, MA: Academic Press; 2008.

[26] NRC. Measuring lead exposure in infants, children, and other sensitive populations. Washington, DC: The National Academies Press; 1993.

[27] CDC. Preventing lead poisoning in young children: a statement by the Centers for Disease Control. Atlanta, GA; 1991.

[28] Dixon SL, Gaitens JM, Jacobs DE, Strauss W, Nagaraja J, Pivetz T, et al. Exposure of U.S. children to residential dust lead, 1999–2004: II. The contribution of lead-contaminated dust to children's blood lead levels. Environ Health Perspect 2009;117:468–74.

[29] US EPA. Framework for cumulative risk assessment, EPA/600/P-02/001F. Washington, DC: U.S. Environmental Protection Agency; 2003.

[30] US EPA. General principles for performing aggregate exposure and risk assessments. Washington, DC: U.S. Environmental Protection; 2001.

[31] US Congress. Food Quality Protection Act of 1996. Public Law 104-170-August 3; 1996 Available at: http://www.gpo.gov/fdsys/pkg/STATUTE-84/pdf/STATUTE-84-Pg1676.pdf.

[32] Olson DA, Corsi RL. In-home formation and emissions of trihalomethanes: the role of residential dishwashers. J Expo Anal Environ Epidemiol 2004;14:109–19.

[33] Weisel CP, Jo WK, Lioy P. Utilization of breath analysis for exposure and dose estimates of chloroform. J Expo Anal Environ Epidemiol 1992;2:55−70.

[34] US EPA. Integrated review plan for the national ambient air quality standards for particulate matter, EPA 452/R-08-004, ORD. Washington, DC: U.S. Environmental Protection Agency; 2008.

[35] Lioy PJ, Weisel CP, Millette JR, Eisenreich S, Vallero D, Offenberg J, et al. Characterization of the dust/smoke aerosol that settled east of the World Trade Center (WTC) in Lower Manhattan after the collapse of the WTC 11 September 2001. Environ Health Perspect 2002;110:703−14.

[36] US EPA. Air quality criteria for particulate matter, EPA/600/P-99/002bF. Research Triangle Park, NC: U.S. Environmental Protection Agency; 2004.

[37] Freeman NC, Ettinger A, Berry M, Rhoads G. Hygiene- and food-related behaviors associated with blood lead levels of young children from lead-contaminated homes. J Expo Anal Environ Epidemiol 1997;7:103−18.

[38] Xue J, Zartarian V, Moya J, Freeman N, Beamer P, Black K, et al. A meta-analysis of children's hand-to-mouth frequency data for estimating nondietary ingestion exposure. Risk Anal 2007;27:411−20.

[39] NRC. Science and decisions: advancing risk assessment. Washington, DC: The National Academies Press; 2009.

[40] Freeman NC, Jimenez M, Reed KJ, Gurunathan S, Edwards RD, Roy A, et al. Quantitative analysis of children's microactivity patterns: the Minnesota children's pesticide exposure study. J Expo Anal Environ Epidemiol 2001;11:501−9.

[41] Reed KJ, Jimenez M, Freeman NCG, Lioy PJ. Quantification of children's hand and mouthing activities through a videotaping methodology. J Expo Anal Environ Epidemiol 1999;9:513−20.

[42] Lioy PJ. Employing dynamical and chemical processes for contaminant mixtures outdoors to the indoor environment: the implications for total human exposure analysis and prevention. J Expo Anal Environ Epidemiol 2006;16:207−24.

[43] Weschler C, Nazaroff WW. SVOC partitioning between the gasphase and settled dirt indoors. Atmos Environ 2010;44:3609−20.

[44] Hamel S, Ellickson K, Lioy PJ. The estimation of the bioaccessibiliy of heavy metals in soils using artifical biofluids to novel methods: mass balance and soil recapture. J Sci Total Environ 1999;243/244:273−83.

[45] Ruby MV, Davis A, Link TE, Schoof R, Chaney RL, Freeman GB, et al. Development of an in vitro screening test to evaluate the in vivo bioacessibility of ingested mine-waste lead. J Environ Sci Technol 1993;27:2870−6.

[46] Fenske RA, Curry PB, Wandelmaier F, Ritter L. Development of dermal and respiratory sampling procedures for human exposure to pesticides in indoor environments. J Expo Anal Environ Epidemiol 1991;1:11−30.

[47] Freeman NCG, Hore P, Black K, Jimenez M, Sheldon L, Tulve N, et al. Contributions of children's activities to pesticide hand loadings following residential pesticide application. J Expo Anal Environ 2004.

[48] Lioy PJ. Assessing total human exposure to contaminants. A multidisciplinary approach. Environ Sci Technol 1990;24:938−45.

CHAPTER 4

Exposure Science Applications and Uses

4.1 EXPOSURE AND ENVIRONMENTAL SCIENCE

Many research studies are now designed to assess the processes and levels of toxicants associated with single or multiple routes and pathways of exposure. The role of traditional environmental science in this process, the left side of Figure 1.1, describes how contaminants are released, transported, and accumulated in the environment and includes many different subfields of investigation for measurements and modeling [1–5]. These areas of research and surveillance support the acquisition of information on the emissions from ambient sources of environmental pollutants, indoor sources, the transport and accumulation of pollutants in environmental media, and the chemical, biological, and physical transformations that can occur in the environment to produce secondary or degradation products. Most environmental science investigations and programs stop at this point in data acquisition and report results and information on environmental quality, compliance with standards and other guidelines, and environmental fate of materials. However, as mentioned previously, when risk assessors use environmental data to complete exposure assessments, the potential exists for the results to have large uncertainties and/or misclassification of exposures. The acceptance of risk assessments in the absence of an evaluation of whether reported environmental levels actually contact individuals or a population has actually been an impediment to exposure science research since these flawed estimates have been used to develop inadequate or incorrect risk management decisions, e.g., ground water pollution issues. To improve risk management decisions, more time needs to be spent to specifically design sampling networks that represent exposure. Suggested basic study designs and the populations or situations that should be used are given in Table 4.1. The results from such studies can be in the forward direction modeling to define the exposure–response relationships or associations, or in the reverse direction modeling to establish exposure to source relationships. Important historical studies have included both internal and external markers [6–9].

Table 4.1 Spatial Considerations: Summary of Sampling Designs and When They Are Most Useful

Sampling Design	Condition for Most Useful Application
Haphazard sampling	Only valid when target population is homogeneous in space and time: hence, not generally recommended
Purposive sampling	Target population well defined and homogeneous, so sample-selection bias is not a problem: or specific environmental samples selected for unique value and interest, rather than for making inferences to wider population
Probability sampling	Homogeneous population
Simple random sampling	
Stratified random sampling	Homogeneous population within strata (subregions); might consider strata as domains of study
Systematic sampling	Frequently most useful; trends over time and space must be quantified
Multistage sampling	Target population large and homogeneous; simple random sampling used to select contiguous groups of population units
Cluster sampling	Economical when population units cluster (e.g., schools of fish); ideally, cluster means are similar in value, but concentrations within clusters should vary widely
Double sampling	Must be strong linear relation between variable of interest and less-expensive or more-easily measured variable

4.2 SOURCE PROXIMITY AND CHARACTERIZING EXPOSURE

4.2.1 Industrial Emissions

The emissions strength, pathway, or transport of contaminants through the environment, and the proximity of sources to people need to be defined to assess the relative importance of environmental emissions on exposure. Industrial releases and mobile source emissions into the atmosphere, water or soil typically are the largest releases into the environment and are the most commonly regulated emissions. Further, the transformation products associated with reactions that include the emitted materials need to be considered in exposure characterizations. However, human exposure analyses allow us to understand the importance of industrial or mobile source emissions relative to other sources of toxic agents. The environmental concentrations resulting from industrial emissions can be determined by different approaches including, but not limited to, release inventories combined with emission modeling, modeling based on mass balance considerations and monitoring measurements either on-site or off-site of the industrial plant. Industrial releases into the ambient air are generally point or line source emissions and well tested mathematical models have been developed to describe their concentration based on meteorological conditions, terrain, and knowledge about the emission characteristics. The assumptions used to develop a particular model, however, must be considered when applying the model to a specific situation. One consideration is whether the receptor of interest is close or more distant from the source since mixing of pollutants within the atmosphere is more efficient and wind effects due to the local topography smaller as pollutants are transported longer distances. The surface water concentration associated with industrial emissions can be estimated from emission rates and water flow. Releases into the soil can be assessed by measurements if there is information available on stability and contaminants removal rate due to leaching and degradation. Additional considerations for evaluating the appropriateness of the exposure estimate from industrial emissions are: (1) whether there is a chronic or acute exposure, (2) the types and degree to which contaminant transformation occurs within the environment, and (3) time frame and multimedia considerations for emissions (e.g., does an air emission deposit on a surface that is used for growing crops so the agent ends up in a food supply). Finally, have processes or regulations changed with time. The latter can influence the significance and interpretation of historic trends.

For nonreactive airborne chemicals, attempts have been made to define a qualitative indicator of potential exposure called the intake fraction. It is defined as the ratio of the total mass inhaled divided by the total mass emitted by a source and can be used as an indicator of the importance of indoor or outdoor air pollution sources on exposure. Based upon proximity of the source to the human receptor, there is a rule of 1000; this means that for inhalation intake, 1 g of indoor emission is roughly equivalent to 1000 g of outdoor emissions in terms of intake of mass. More details on the intake fraction have been published in a review by Bennett et al. [10].

4.2.2 Mobile Source Emissions

Mobile source emissions (on road and off road vehicles) have been recently identified as important contributors to air pollutants in urban settings. Emissions include volatile organic compounds present in or added to petroleum products to increase the efficiency of the engine and reduce emission of specific gases (e.g., carbon monoxide) and fine/ultrafine particulate matter levels that result from high-temperature combustion. The impact of mobile source emissions on respiratory ailments, particularly in children and the elderly, and cardiovascular effects, in the elderly and individuals with preexisting conditions, has been well documented and used in standard setting. A review of the problem indicates that exposures near major roadways or congestion near schools and neighborhoods can be a major concern. Urban planning has failed to take near field contacts into consideration since proximity of congested and major and expanding roadway to schools continues to increase and has resulted in higher children's exposures to mobile source emissions [11]. This is in spite of the major advances that have been made in automobile emission control over the past 40 years in the United States and elsewhere. Generally, mobile source air pollution has decreased, but there continues to be hot spots of air pollution related to mobile source emissions. This has led to the examination of exposure associated with urban air pollution in well-defined locations called "Hot Spots" [12].

4.2.3 Personal and Home Products

In contrast to industrial and mobile sources emissions, emissions from personal and home products will release relatively small quantities of pollutants from a single source (e.g., disinfection spray or deodorizer) [11,13,14]. However, due to their proximity to people or the releases being in an enclosed area (indoors), where dilution occurs at a slower rate than in the ambient environment, these emissions can have a relatively high percent contribution to total personal exposure. This supports the idea of a high intake fraction and higher inhalation contact, and contributions to other exposure routes because of adsorption and deposition. Considerations associated with contacts caused by personal and home product emissions include: (1) understanding the active and "inert" agents in the product, (2) how the product is actually used and not just the suggested label use, (3) whether or not the components are altered with time or accumulate within the indoor environment, and (4) whether or not reactions occur indoors and on surfaces. The impact of home and personal products on exposure to pollutants is also a reflection of the large percentage of time that individuals spend within the home environments and the manner that agents are in contact with an individual. Further, with the introduction of nanoparticle technology, a new species of pollutant is being released in the indoor and personal environment, and the number of products is expanding significantly each day [15,16]. A true population exposure study that can guide the toxicology is essential, since most current toxicology studies are focusing on the pure substance or initial products and not the form of the nanoparticle that actually contacts the consumer.

4.2.4 Commercial Emissions

Individuals are exposed to toxic agents from commercial businesses (e.g., drycleaners, gasoline stations, auto body shops). This occurs when visiting these establishments to purchase products or using their services, when transporting items purchased, when using the purchased items, (with the latter being related to exposures to personal and home products), or when in contact with ambient emissions from the facility. There can be large variations in exposure to toxicants across a population, which is dependent upon the proximity of one's residence to the commercial source and activities related to the items introduced into commerce. For example, a major concern in the 1990s was trichloroethylene and tetrachloroethylene emissions from dry cleaning facilities in cities [17].

4.2.5 Hazardous Waste Emissions

Potential exposure to contaminants present in hazardous wastes depends upon whether the wastes are still in a publicly accessible location designated as a hazardous waste site or the hazardous material has migrated off-site into a local neighborhood. Since hazardous wastes by definition have toxic substances, determining the exposure to the population is the key component in the risk evaluation. Typically the hazard can be defined through multicompound toxicity and exposures studies. Activities that can lead to contact must also be determined for each situation. Migration of wastes off-site increases the potential exposure to individuals in the surrounding community and can occur through the air if the pollutants are volatile or present in dust or soil that can be blown off-site and via groundwater from leaching. Besides modeling or measuring the levels off-site, determining how people may contact the toxic agent can be estimated by assessment of the activity and behavior of people in the area. The activities leading to exposure vary with different age groups since children, teenagers, adults, and the elderly are likely to have different activity patterns. This is not different from how to address the exposure issues associated with each of the preceding sources, but there is a prescribed method available for addressing local population contact with emissions from hazardous waste sites [18].

Consideration should be given as to whether access to the site occurs and by whom and the degree to which agents are distributed to the soil of the surrounding area. Such distribution of material can lead to potential exposure while community members are outdoors, from track-in of materials into homes, or contamination of public or private drinking water supplies. Many hazardous waste sites have a plethora of toxins that includes trace metals (e.g., lead, cadmium, arsenic), organic solvents (e.g., chlorinated solvents, benzene), and semivolatile organic compounds (e.g., PCBs, pesticides).

4.3 EXPOSURE AND ENVIRONMENTAL HEALTH SCIENCES

The right side of Figure 1.1 includes toxicology, a scientific discipline in which investigators conduct mechanistic and toxicity testing research on toxic or suspected toxic agents. That part of the continuum also includes environmental and occupational epidemiology and clinical medicine disciplines which involve developing an understanding of the etiology of diseases caused by toxic agents, including hypotheses and/or diagnoses that link toxic agent exposures to specific health outcomes. The three fields—epidemiology, clinical investigation, and clinical intervention—benefit most directly from exposure science research and applications since they are associated with analyses of human populations. However, in many cases, epidemiologic studies have attempted to demonstrate an exposure–response relationship by collecting a minimal amount of exposure data and employing environmental measures, survey data, or guesses as surrogates of exposure (e.g., violations of standards and spatial proximity). Exposure misclassification can lead to underestimation or overestimation of the actual risk or not provide the data needed to identify an association between an environmental toxicant and an adverse health effect [19–21].

Ultimately, risk management benefits directly from modern exposure characterization since its results can be used to reduce the uncertainties in the application of control strategies or source identification compared to relying on environmental quality data [11,22]. Thus, exposure scientists are essential for increasing the likelihood that (1) meaningful exposure–response relationships or associations can be established, (2) source to exposure relationships can be defined, and (3) eventually approaches can be designed to reduce risk and/or explain the occurrence of a suspected environmental or occupational health-related outcome.

When reviewing information to relate a source to exposure to affect relationship, it would be valuable to start by determining how well a source or proximate source can be linked by one or more pathways and routes of exposure. The exposure route and magnitude would then be evaluated as to ascertain if they could lead to a health outcome. Establishing the linkages among source–exposure–effect in the initial evaluation of a project can improve the design of epidemiologic studies and improve clinical interventions.

4.4 EXPOSURE SCIENCE AND CAUSATION

Establishing the presence or absence of human "contact" with toxic agents is necessary for showing causation or at least strengthens associations identified in an epidemiological investigation. The results from exposure measurements can define the association between the intensity and temporal characteristic of the exposure and the biology of the disease and provide information to mitigate a source or end exposure within the population or to an individual at risk [21]. The results from exposure science studies also can improve the selection of the levels of a chemical or other agent of concern used in mitigation studies. The use of "*in vitro* tools" can provide more rapid results for improving the hazard portion of risk assessment [23,24]. These should be used in conjunction with the introduction of new sensors to improve multiroute exposure characterization [11].

4.5 EXPOSURE SCIENCE AND THE LAW

The application of exposure science to litigation and other legal actions starts with the desire to attest to or refute a hypothesized exposure-health response relationship. Critical components needed to achieve such an understanding are the documentation of the potential presence or absence of causality between the toxic agent and the health effect (which typically is based on toxicological, clinical, or epidemiological evidence) and evidence documenting the contact or lack of contact with a toxic agent by the individual or population in question (exposure science evidence). If contact is established, the next steps are to estimate the magnitude and duration of the exposure to determine if that is sufficient to cause the adverse outcome. This is necessary in toxic tort cases to effectively assess liability of a defendant in a situation where a plaintiff is suing for damages to his/her health, or the health of family members or a group in a class action claim. Legal actions to protect consumers are usually brought by groups including NGOs, affected industries, and less frequently by members of the public. In recent years, these efforts have been expanded to populations at risk who identify local problems. They may not know the problems exactly but can have significant information needed to design a study intervention to protect their community from environmental exposures [11].

Other areas where exposure science is necessary are formulation of a national environmental or occupational health standard control strategy, development or updating state/local regulation to protect human health, and safety standards used to protect our food supply or consumer products from contaminants. Food and consumer product standards on a global scale are relatively new areas that have been of increasing concern because of the global economy and the lack of standards or oversight in some manufacturing facilities and food production in some countries.

REFERENCES

[1] Lioy PJ. Assessing total human exposure to contaminants. A multidisciplinary approach. Environ Sci Technol 1990;24:938–45.

[2] Zartarian V, Bahadori T, McKone TE. Adoption of an offical ISEA glossary. J Expo Anal Environ Epidemiol 2005;15:1–5.

[3] Duan N. Models for human exposure to air pollution. Environ Int 1982;8:305–9.

[4] Mckone TE. Human exposure to chemicals from multiple media and through multiple pathways—research overview and comments. Risk Anal 1991;11:5–10.

[5] Mckone TE, Daniels JI. Estimating human exposure through multiple pathways from Air, Water, and Soil. Regulatory Toxicol Pharm 1991;13:36–61.

[6] Pellizzari E, Lioy PJ, Quackenboss J, Whitmore R, Clayton A, Freeman N, et al. Population-based exposure measurements in EPA region 5: a phase I field study in support of the national human exposure assessment survey. J Expo Anal Environ Epidemiol 1995;5:583.

[7] Dixon SL, Gaitens JM, Jacobs DE, Strauss W, Nagaraja J, Pivetz T, et al. Exposure of U.S. Children to Residential Dust Lead, 1999–2004: II. The contribution of lead-contaminated dust to children's blood lead levels. Environ Health Perspect 2009;117:468–74.

[8] Hore P, Robson M, Freeman N, Zhang J, Wartenberg D, Ozkaynak H, et al. Chlorpyrifos accumulation patterns for child-accessible surfaces and objects and urinary metabolite excretion by children for 2 weeks after crack-and-crevice application. Environ Health Perspect 2005;113:211–9.

[9] Egehy PP, Cohen Hubal EA, Tulve N, Melnyk LJ, Morgan MK, Fortmann R, et al. Review of pesticide urinary biomarker measurements from selected US EPA children's observational exposure studies. Int J Res Public Health 2011;8:1727–54.

[10] Bennett DH, McKone TE, Evans JS, Nazaroff WW, Margni MD, Jolliet O, et al. Defining intake fraction. Environ Sci Technol 2002;36:206A−11A.

[11] NRC. Exposure science in the 21st century: a vision and a strategy. Washington, DC: The National Academies Press; 2012.

[12] Zhu X, Fan Z-H, Wu X, Meng Q, Wang S-W, Tang X, et al. Spatial variation of volatile organic compounds in a "Hot Spot" for air pollution. Atmos Environ 2008;42:7329−39.

[13] Lioy PJ. Exposure science: a view of the past and milestones for the future. Environ Health Perspect 2010;118:1081−90.

[14] Spengler J, Samet JM, McCarthy JF. Indoor air quality handbook. New York, NY: McGraw Hill; 2000.

[15] Lioy PJ, Nazarenko Y, Han TW, Lioy MJ, Mainelis G. Nanotechnology and exposure science what is needed to fill the research and data gaps for consumer products. Int J Occup Environ Health 2010;16:378−87.

[16] Nazarenko Y, Zhen H, Han T, Lioy PJ, Mainelis G. Nanomaterial inhalation exposure from nanotechnology-based cosmetic powders: a quantitative assessment. J Nanopart Res 2012;14:1229.

[17] Schreiber JS. An exposure and risk assessment regarding the presence of tetrachlorethene in human breast milk. J Expo Anal Environ Epidemiol 1992;2:15−26.

[18] US EPA. Guidelines for exposure assessment. EPA/600/Z-92/001. Washington, DC: U.S. Environmental Protection, Risk Assessment Forum; 1992.

[19] Lebowitz M, Lioy PJ, McKone TE, Spengler J, Adgate JL, Bennett D, et al. The necessity of observing children's exposure of contaminants in their real-world environmental settings; 2008.

[20] US EPA. Integrated review plan for the national ambient air quality standards for particulate matter. EPA 452/R-08-004, ORD. Washington, DC: U.S. Environmental Protection Agency; 2008.

[21] US EPA. Air quality criteria for particulate matter. EPA/600/P-99/002bF. Research Triangle Park, NC: U.S. Environmental Protection; 2004.

[22] NRC. Science and decisions: advancing risk assessment. Washington, DC: The National Academies Press; 2009.

[23] Cohen-Hubal EA. Biologically relevant exposure science for 21st century toxicity testing. Toxicol Sci 2009;111:226−32.

[24] NRC. Toxicity testing in the 21st century: a vision and a strategy. Washington, DC: The National Academies Press; 2007.

—

CHAPTER 5

Exposure Science Research Design

The design of exposure science investigations takes many forms, as outlined in the 1991 NRC report. The two most common designs are "Purposive Sampling" and "Probability Sampling." For the former, the "target population" is well defined and many times homogeneous (with controls if possible), or involves collection of specific samples to evaluate unique exposure or health questions (see Table 4.1). These convenience samples can limit the ability to make inferences about wider populations but provide inputs for exposure modeling or address exposures from a suspected source [1]. However, in each design, biases may occur because of the method of population or location selection. Probability sampling is derived from statistical sampling designs which include random, systematic, stratified, and other (e.g., cluster, multistage) sampling protocols (see Table 4.1). These measure exposures that are representative of the larger population the sampled individuals were selected from. However, if the numbers of samples collected are small, while they could provide a good estimate of the mean exposure they may miss the extremes in exposure which often drive the health risk.

The key component of each human exposure study design is the measurement or estimation of contact with toxic agents. Two approaches have been developed to measure exposure based on the time-dependent nature of exposure: direct and indirect methods. Both methods have added complications compared to traditional environmental measurements which can often be accomplished by placing monitors in locations where access is controlled by the team collecting the sample. Unless the concentrations where the samples are collected and where different groups of people actual spend their time are the same, these samples would not be representative of the contaminant exposure concentrations For example, does a roof top provide an adequate measure of exposure to carbon monoxide from street traffic [2], are the toxic agent levels in food market baskets the same as the levels in the food a person consumes, or are the levels measured in a groundwater aquifer measured two miles from a home similar to the levels found in that home's well water [3].

Some environmental measurements can be used to estimate exposure and are employed quite frequently in developing exposure profiles for large populations. This has worked for fine particulate matter ($PM_{2.5}$), which is a ubiquitous air pollutant that can have a long lifetime in the atmosphere [4]. In other situations where one is trying to reconstruct exposures to an agent from very specific sources affecting an individual or a limited population, the exposures may be unique enough for quantitative information on environmental levels to be sufficient to construct the intensity of contact and risk to members of the general population [5].

Collection of samples for characterization of exposure using the direct measurement method requires coordination with the individuals or populations being evaluated so that samples can be collected in locations, media encountered or items consumed that are relevant to the study population. This can be a burden on the participants but can lead to meaningful community participation. Determination of historic exposures can be challenging when conditions have changed and current measurements do not reflect past levels. Historic exposure characterization requires an understanding of the activity patterns of the individuals at the time of the exposure, a mechanism for employing either measured concentrations under similar conditions or an exposure model developed using the specific scenarios. The community can be an important source of information documenting what may have changed over time. Exposure characterizations of specific source emissions quite frequently are used to establish environmental exposure–response relationships and require many measurements to augment environmental monitoring data [1,6–8].

The direct method for measuring exposure uses personal monitoring or biological monitoring of individuals [9]. Measurements of exposure are made with varying degrees of regularity in workplaces, primarily directed toward achieving compliance with federal OSHA or Mine Safety regulations [10]. The following are key components needed to assess each exposure route: (1) for environmental inhalation exposures, an individual would continuously wear an air monitor; (2) for dietary ingestion, exposure measurement of levels in food and beverage samples that match what a person ate along with quantity and frequency of the items consumed; (3) for nondietary ingestion exposure measurement, determine the amount of the contaminants on items placed in the mouth, including hands, or the surfaces hands contact along with the frequency of hand or object to mouth activities; and (4) for dermal exposure, wearing of patches, hand wipe samples and measurement of water concentrations used for washing, showering, bathing, and swimming along with information of the frequency and durations of those activities.

Biomonitoring provides a measurement of the body burden of toxic chemical compounds, elements, or their metabolites in a biological matrix that is proportional to the exposure. More details on methods to collect personal samples and biological monitoring are provided in subsequent sections of this chapter.

The second measurement approach is indirect exposure monitoring. This method usually defines locations or activities where uniform exposure concentrations occur and takes samples from those locations which are then used in combination with the frequency and duration that an individual is in that location or activity in Eq. (2.2) to characterize exposure. The use of microenvironmental sampling is the more common approach in conducting exposure monitoring.

5.1 HUMAN ACTIVITIES AND BEHAVIOR

As discussed throughout the book, a major difference between exposure research and traditional environment science studies is the need to collect human behavior and time activity information. The emphasis that regulatory and public health agencies have placed on collection of environmental data alone may suggest that those measurements are the most important component for analyses of exposure. While they are a crucial component of characterizing exposure, they represent only one of the many tools. Two additional critical components of exposure are characterization of human activity patterns and human behaviors. Each can alter a person's exposure to toxicants. Research on this critical aspect of exposure science began in the 1980s with the documentation by different research teams of common activities which appeared to enhance or reduce exposure [10−21]. These data were primarily obtained using the principles of survey research, but using questions focused primarily on locations, time spent in various locations, and the activities performed in each location. The answers obtained help define contact with toxic agents. Other information collected in exposure questionnaires are concerned with potential sources of contaminants that exist in specific locations, and general characteristics of the home or workplace environment [10–12]. The questionnaires data have been incorporated in nationwide computer-ized information systems on human activities which have led to the production of the national database established by the EPA, called Consolidated Human Activity Database (CHAD) [14]. It is critical that these types of databases are continually updated to reflect ever-evolving activities and behaviors across different segments of the population. CHAD and other databases are now used extensively in exposure models and to estimate exposure for single and multiple routes of entry into the body. However, some of the information on activity patterns related to the intensity and duration of contact with a toxicant and ultimately the exposure still has large uncertainties, e.g., a mother spraying toys with antibacterial chemicals or adult using vola-tile toxicants in an unventilated home workshop. Examples of recent changes in behavior and activity patterns that need to be incorporated in databases are the wide use of cell phones, laptop computers, and now smart phones with many "apps." Serendipitously, this has led to the development of novel types of research to fill in this major gap in knowledge, including the use of smart phones for acquisition of space and source data over time [6,22].

Investigators have used questionnaires to quantify types of beha-viors that affect exposure, though sometimes with large uncertainties. For example, questionnaires completed by parents and caregivers provided estimates of the number of times children contacted surfaces and then put their hands in their mouth during an hour were well below 10 per hour. Subsequent observational studies have documented that young children have a much higher rate of hand to mouth contact after touching surfaces.

For water, questionnaires need to be completed to obtain informa-tion on the amount of tap water consumed and the results need to be compared to bottled water consumption in a community. If only bottled water is consumed, then basing the exposure to toxic agents in the tap water would overestimate the exposure.

While epidemiological investigations still use questionnaires, the questions are now much better phrased in an attempt to better capture the behaviors that influence exposure. More accurate human behavioral information has improved the data used to interpret microenvironmental data for reconstructing or predicting potentially hazardous exposure (e.g., attached garages). One of the best methods available for improving exposure estimates has been observational research studies conducted in a manner that does not alter the participant's behavior. One way this has been accomplished is by videotaping children and adults in their "daily" world after obtaining appropriate consent from the participants, parents, and the Institutional Review Board (IRB) for human subjects. The individual doing the videotaping needed to be unobtrusive and not interact with the subjects. This tool was first employed to evaluate the frequency of hands touching surfaces to estimate the number of times a child contacted surfaces sprayed with pesticides [18−20]. The approach has reduced uncertainties in exposure estimates for many different types of populations, especially toddlers and active youths. For instance, young children can have hand surface touching to mouth transfers of up to 40 times per hours. At the same time, the research has opened a window for exposure into the world of children's behaviors. Unexpected behaviors were observed that can lead to high exposures. These included children sitting on top of containers containing hazardous substances, playing in open pesticide treated crop fields, and chewing on many types of surfaces and objects. Observational tools have been instrumental in validating the distribution of values that are inputted into exposure models. It is critical to determine the validity of the input values used in exposure models to accurately estimate exposure, which greatly improves the evaluation of environmental health problems.

5.2 EXTRAPOLATION OF ENVIRONMENTAL QUALITY DATA TO EXPOSURE DATA

The continuum, Figure 1.1, is the starting point for determining whether or not an exposure can or has occurred, and identifying the information available to define source to exposure relationships. The first term in the continuum is the source since without emissions into the ambient environment, home, school, workplace, or other microenvironment/activity a person engages in there will be no toxicant present to contact or an exposure. As mentioned in Chapters 2 and 4, the word source usually produces images of an industrial stack effluent pipe on a large tract of land that is surrounded by a fence, or the emissions from the tailpipe of a motor vehicle. These are typically large environmental sources, but in terms of the modern applications of exposure science

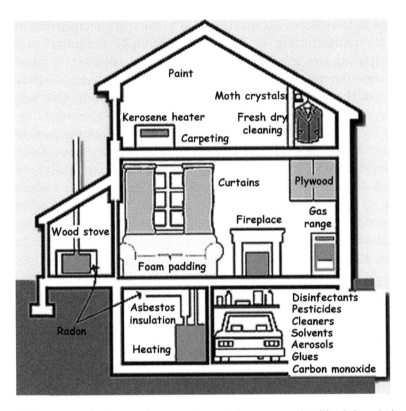

Figure 5.1 Source categories that contribute to multi-route indoor exposures. http://dec.alaska.gov/air/anpms/ id_aq/idaqhome.htm.

versus environmental science there are many smaller emission sources, e.g., gasoline stations, tap water, dry cleaned clothing, or even products used in homes, that can be more important contributors to the total exposure for specific agents. This occurs when small sources are in close proximity to an individual for a sufficient duration. Figure 5.1 portrays some obvious and subtle sources that exist within a home. Some examples of important sources are found in Table 5.1. Identifying "proximate" sources is an important component in solving a problem or conducting forensic exposure investigation. Thus, the investigations of causal relationships (exposure–response) have to consider many sources beyond the most obvious or traditional. Box 5.1 provides an example of how different microenvironments contribute to benzene exposures.

Box 5.2 provides an example of how rugs and carpets can contribute to pesticide exposure in homes calculated using data from Morgan et al. [26] and the Exposure Factors Handbook.

Table 5.1 Proximate Sources That Contribute to Personal Exposures

Location	Media	Contaminants
Home	Rugs/Carpets Dust tracked in on shoes, pets	Dust, semivolatile organic compounds, e.g., pesticides; metals, e.g., lead; allergens; molds; and bacteria
	New home furnishings, Paint Tap water—chlorinated, contaminated well water	Volatile organic compounds (VOC) (e.g., formaldehyde), chloroform, solvents
	Combustion sources: cigarettes, wood stoves, and fireplaces	Particles, polyaromatic hydrocarbons
	Gas appliances: stoves, heaters	Nitrogen dioxide
	Inadequate maintenance or cleaning: peeling paint, humid/moist area, water leakage	Lead from old paint, mold growth, allergens, pet dander, dust mite
Personal care products	Sprayed, released, applied directly on body	Nanoparticles: phthalates, formaldehyde, parabens, triclosan (endocrine disruptors)
Home cleaning products	Sprayed and used on surfaces throughout the home	Ammonia, 1,4 dioxane, alkylphenol ethoxylates, 2-butoxyethanol, chlorinated solvents, petroleum-based chemicals, chlorine bleach
Indoor air chemistry	Reactions with ozone, nitrogen dioxide, nitrites, chlorine with home products (e.g., air fresheners), and emissions from people	Aldehydes, ketones, chloramine, nitrosamines from reaction with limonene, pinene, diethanolamine
Pesticides	Sprayed in/around home by residents and commercial applicators	Pyrethroids often redistributed throughout the home and into foam in toys, furnishing, carpets
Automobile cabin	Poorly maintained vehicle	Gasoline VOC
	Refuel at gasoline station in heavy traffic	Diesel particles
Attached garage	Gas can, small gas engines, automobiles	Gasoline VOC, e.g., benzene, methyl *tert*-butyl ether, hexane
Public modes of transportation	Bus, train, bicycle near traffic, airplane	Diesel emissions, CO, ozone, bacteria, viruses, aldehydes
Outside play area	Backyard, artificial turf fields	Lead deposited from previous lead-gas emission or exterior paint, pesticide applied to grass, color agent on artificial turf

5.2.1 Multimedia Concentrations

Many toxicants whose exposures can significantly affect human health can be present simultaneously in multiple media. The primary media of concern for exposure are the air, water, soil, dust, and food. In some situations, the contaminant is present in multiple media all of which will be a public health concern, while in other situations only

Box 5.1 Benzene Exposures: a Multisource Example

The volatile organic compound, benzene, has been a major concern for human health effects since the industrial revolution. Its presence in gasoline results in many potential exposure pathways that include: leaking underground gasoline storage tanks which can contaminate water sources, contaminated soil gas that penetrates the basement of home, vapors emitted from gasoline cans and small gasoline engines (e.g., lawn mowers, snow blowers) stored in a garage attached to a home, and evaporative releases from poorly maintained automobiles. Benzene vapors can also be released during the fueling of a vehicle or the inappropriate use of gasoline indoors as a solvent to remove grease. Benzene is also a component of cigarette smoke, so, smokers and individuals breathing environmental tobacco smoke have additional inhalation benzene exposure. Emissions from each can yield higher benzene exposures where people live, play, or congregate than from current industrial releases.

Benzene exposure was calculated using Eq. (2.2) for an average nonsmoking adult (data from Weisel [23] and the Exposure Factors Handbook [24]):

Microenvironment	Air Concentration ($\mu g/m^3$)	Duration (min) in Microenvironment	Daily Exposure	Percent Contribution (%)
Indoor residence	4.9	946	4600	37
Outdoor	3.1	187	580	5
Indoor other	1.4	211	3000	24
In transit	24	93	2200	18
Refueling	700	3	2100	16

one medium will be of concern. Further, the persistence of a contaminant at concentrations of concern may not be the same within each medium. These situations usually are studied using approaches associated with cumulative and aggregated exposures.

Lead is an example of a multimedia pollutant [27]. It is emitted into the air from point sources, e.g., smelter, and will be present at the highest air concentrations at the point of emission with the levels varying with time as a function of variations in the emission rate and the local meteorology. Historically, the highest widespread atmospheric levels in the United States have been associated with lead emissions from automobiles, until lead was banned from gasoline in 1996. The subsequent atmospheric deposition of lead is contributed to

Box 5.2 Carpets as Reservoir for Dust

Rugs and carpets in the home have been identified as a proximate source that cuts across many typical chemical, physical, or biological toxicants. Carpets and rugs are used to keep a home: warm, quiter, esthetically pleasing, and to prevent injury, etc. However, there is an "unintended consequence" (a term that is referred to frequently as we try to replace toxic agents with presumably less toxic agents) from using carpets. That is accumulation of microscopic levels of nonvolatile and semivolatile materials and biological active materials over time. These materials may be toxic and may not quickly degrade. Pesticides sources in the home include routine pest control applications and transport into the home through the air from field and crop applications (sometimes called drift). Pesticides can also be tracked inside on shoes that have been in contact with outdoor areas that have been treated with pesticides or on domestic animals. Once indoors, pesticides can redistribute on toys and accumulate in the dust in carpets [25].

Internal exposures across different routes for *trans*-permethrin (pesticides) for a 3−6 years old calculated using Eq. (3.2) data from Morgan et al. [26] and the Exposure Factors Handbook [24].

	Media Concentration	Intake Amount	Internal Exposure (ng/day)	Percent
Dust (ingestion)	300 ng/g	50 mg/day	15	34
Soil (ingestion)	3.0 ng/g	60 mg/day	0.18	0.4
Food (ingestion)	0.22 ng/g	110 g/day	24	54
Inhalation	0.32 ng/m^3	12 m^3/day	3.4	8
Dermal	0.01 ng/cm^2	1.5% absorption 80-cm^2 hand area 120 contacts/day	1.4	3

soil concentrations. Lead deposited in soil will remain prevalent in an area until all top soil is cleaned up either by removal and replacement by a clean fill or covering by sufficient layer of clean top soil so it will not be exposed again. Lead from exterior paint in homes built prior to 1978, particularly prior to 1950, which crumbles, peels, or chalks, contributes to lead in the soil near homes and can present an exposure pathway to children playing. A second medium that contributed to lead exposure is drinking water. Lead can originate with the water source, during water treatment, within the public or private distribution system or within the pipes in a home. It leaches into tap water from older lead pipes and plumbing solder and fittings. Thus, lead can build up in concentration in water when it sits in pipes and plumbing fixtures for extended time periods. This result in elevated ingestion of lead when water that sits overnight in the water pipes in a home is consumed (known as the first flush) the next day. Letting water run for a while to flush the water from home pipes typically reduces lead exposures. Another step that can be taken to reduce exposure from water contaminants is to use a properly maintained water purifier for water used for drinking and/or cooking. Information on activity patterns (tap water and bottled water use) and house characteristics (use, type, and maintenance of filters) are needed to determine lead exposure from tap water. Lead in the general food supply is typically low and sporadic, but additional sources of lead could be: found in vegetables growing in contaminated soil, accumulate during the preparation, or food eaten after placing on dusty surfaces in the home. Children and adults will pick up food that has fallen on the floor or other surfaces and consume it. These include sticky items (e.g., lollipops) or food wet with saliva. Those food items and unwashed hands can result in lead ingestion exposure from accumulated dust. A medium that contributes to nonfood ingestion of lead is paint in some homes built prior to 1978, particularly prior to the 1950s. If lead-based paint chips are present, there is a potential high exposure to lead if the paint chips end up on hands, particularly of children. Lead is occasionally present in the glaze and paint of pottery, used in some cosmetics, as a dye or pigment in some cultural activities and recently been identified to be present in brightly colored toys and jewelry. Lead is also used in a number of occupations and can be brought home on the clothing of workers. Elevated blood lead levels in children are one of the major public health problems of our time. However, due to multitude of sources, it can be challenging to identify the actual exposure pathway(s) and source(s) of lead exposure, and many other toxicants.

The above introduced the concept of source emissions and multimedia concentrations that result in aggregate exposure. To achieve contact, a source whether ultimate or proximate must be linked in some way to a route of entry in the body: inhalation, ingestion, dermal, and on occasion injection.

5.3 EXPOSURE MEASUREMENTS

Exposure measurements are optimally conducted by measuring each media that the individual or population contact in each location that could contain the contaminant of interest. Personal monitors can be used for inhalation exposure (see Section 5.3.4).

5.3.1 Questionnaires and Surveys

Questionnaires and surveys are used to assess activities and locations of people that can lead to potential exposures. These instruments can be used to collect information from large numbers of participants prospectively, alone or in combination with microenvironmental sampling, or retrospectively to assess historic exposures. Questionnaires can be administrated in person, by telephone, through web sites and via mail. The design and validation of any questionnaire or survey is critical to obtaining valid exposure information. Questions should be framed in simple, unambiguous, direct, and understandable language to the person answering the question, and in some cases languages other than English. This requires careful choice of wording that avoids technical jargon and uses language the participants would be familiar with. Question format can be open ended, in which the subject completes a response, or closed ended/multiple choice, in which the responder selects one or more responses. For closed-ended questions, all possible answers to the question should be provided ("none of the above" can be a choice) with no overlap between the answer choices. The choices can be individual responses, encompass a range of values or a rating scale. Closed-ended questions are often preferable as they are more compatible with coding and storing of data in computerized form for subsequent statistical analyses.

Prior to developing the questions, the activities and potential sources of the agents of interest and potential confounders for any health effect of concern need to be identified; that is, know how you want to use the results before you start (what is your research question) or you will likely not obtain the information necessary to answer your questions. A common problem is not including all potential sources of the hazards of concern. This could happen if the investigator is not familiar with the culture or residential area of subject population, or not being familiar with potential sources used within or affecting a home or other microenvironment. Two critical components associated with implementing questionnaires are (1) pilot testing and (2) validation studies. After reviewing the questionnaires among the investigators and staff, it should be administrated to a small subpopulation of participants in the target community. Then the team can obtain feedback as to how well the questions are understood and if there are suggestions on a question's wording or additional questions that the participants might suggest as being important. The questionnaire can then be adjusted appropriately prior to administrating it for the full study.

The validation of the responses is equivalent to quality control/quality assurance steps taken in any research project, but it is often very difficult to accomplish when working with human subjects. Two possible approaches are (1) including several questions that inquire about the same information in different sections of the questionnaire but are worded in slightly different fashions and (2) administrating the questionnaire more than once. In each case the answers should be consistent, with the caveat that the responses have not changed with time. Other considerations are responses should be with valid ranges for open-ended questions and the validity of the conclusions drawn from the results are appropriate for the evaluated populations.

Many studies have developed questionnaires to assess exposure and these can serve as the basis for questionnaires needed in future studies [11,28,29]. If the same modules of questions are used, then the responses can be compared across studies. There are many additional considerations when designing questionnaires. The order of questions can be important as earlier questions can influence the response to subsequent questions and the writing style should be consistent. [If ratings are used as choices, they should be in the same order among questions (do not have some lowest to highest and then the next set of questions highest to lowest)]. It is suggested to avoid or leave to the end of the questionnaire the questions that might evoke a charged emotional response or ask about finances. Number the questions and indicate how many questions remain can be helpful to the participants. Finally, do not insert extraneous questions since participants can lose interest in answering long questionnaires.

With the advent of web-based questionnaires, branching algorithms can be used that can skip sections of a questionnaire based on a previous answer indicating that the section is not relevant [30]. This can reduce the time required for its administration. For example on a home questionnaire, if an individual indicates they do not have a garage attached to a home, questions can be skipped about what is stored in an attached garage. Web-based questionnaires can also be written to avoid the participant skipping critical questions by requiring a response before being allowed to answer the next question or entering invalid answers, e.g., limiting an acceptable answer about the age of the subject to values between 0 and 120 years. All individuals who administer the questionnaire should be provided clear, detailed instructions for their doing so and be taught not to lead the participant to a particular answer. The design of a questionnaire and its administration requires training and skills. These should be done in collaboration with experienced practitioners, and all have to be approved by at least a local IRB.

5.3.2 Microenvironments

The concept of microenvironments is a critical component of exposure modeling and estimation for risk assessment. Microenvironments have typically been defined as an individual volume or an aggregate of locations, or even activities within a location. They have a homogeneous concentration of the pollutant being evaluated and can be considered a perfectly mixed or ideal compartment [8]. Thus, a microenvironment is the place where the activities of individuals would have the same exposure even as they move around within the microenvironment. If an individual would move to another location or engage in a different activity in the same location that resulted in a different exposure then that would be considered a different microenvironment. Defining a microenvironment and determining the exposure concentration associated with it is a critical component of exposure modeling. At the simplest level, the microenvironmental concentration data are multiplied by the time spent in that microenvironment which is then summed across the different microenvironments encountered over the time period of interest (see Eq. (2.2)). This approach does not account for variability in exposure intensity caused by different human behaviors that can occur in those microenvironments. The US EPA time activity pattern database, CHAD, lists the frequency and duration that people spend in different microenvironments [14]. A simple listing of typical microenvironments might include outdoors, indoor at residence, indoor at work or school, in transit, and indoor-other. The selection of unique microenvironments that should be considered will vary with the contaminant considered, exposure route, and where and what people do in those locations. For example, exposure to disinfection by-products (DBP) from chlorinated water would include in addition to the five microenvironments listed above, the shower stall and bathroom in the residential indoor microenvironment and swimming pools as a recreational indoor microenvironment because these microenvironments have strong source terms that greatly elevated DBP concentrations there compared to other locations.

5.3.3 Biological Monitoring

A biological marker is a direct measure of an exposure that is a physiological response or a chemical/biochemical measured within body fluids or tissues whose concentration is proportional to the exposure to the agent of concern. Biomarkers of exposure include the parent compound or element, its metabolite or adduct. The theoretical lifetimes of biomarkers in the body are found in Figure 2.1. Clearly, the time course biomarker in the body is weighted by the agent of concern and the nature of the agent or metabolite or adduct. Each will be of importance in determining the significance for long- and short-term biological effects.

The body fluids and tissues in which biomarkers have been measured include breath, blood, urine, hair, finger or toe nails, breast milk, adipose tissue, and nasal lavage. The presence of a biomarker is a confirmation that an exposure has occurred, provided that the biomarker measured is unique to a specific exposure agent. However, many metabolites or responses can be associated with multiple agents which often preclude a definitive statement about whether the external exposure is from a specific agent. In addition, quality assurance/quality control protocols must be used to verify that no contamination of the samples or losses after collection and during storage has occurred, common problems with some biomarker measurements. Biomarkers concentrations typically change in the body with time due to continued metabolism or excretion from the body (see Figure 2.1). The concentration changes often follow an exponential time curve but most measurements are made on samples collected at a single or a limited number of time points. Some of the better documented biomarkers are blood levels of (Polychlorinated Biphenols) PCBs, lead, carbon monoxide, and mercury. Since the mid-1990s, the US Center for

Disease Control and Prevention (CDC) has been routinely measuring many organic compounds and metals as part of the National Health and Nutrition Examination Survey [17,31−33]. These measurements provide information on baseline levels and temporal and spatial trends for the national concentration distributions of over a hundred toxicants. The data can be used to determine whether or not an individual's levels are within the national norms or at the extremes of the distributions. Biomarkers can sometimes provide information on the dose storage in the body, and the route of entry into the body. Genetic polymorphisms in metabolic enzymes or phenotypes that induce or suppress metabolism can alter the rate of change in the biomarker concentration resulting in potential large interindividual differences in the biomarker levels from the same exposure [29,34−39]. However, biomarker measurements in isolation of information about sources of exposure do not provide enough information for determining when, where, how, and the magnitude of the exposure. Further, in the absence of human activity data they are not informative about the true source of the exposure. The full use of biomarkers information to potentially evaluate pharmacokinetic and pharmacodynamic changes in the body requires information about the time frame of the exposure and route. Thus highlighting the need for obtaining measurements of both internal and external markers of exposures.

5.3.4 Personal Monitoring

Measurements of personal exposure are made to characterize pollutant levels at an individual as a direct measure of contact [6,8,9,38]. For inhalation exposure, the inlet for the sampler or monitor is placed in the breathing zone of the individual. The two most common inhalation samplers are active and passive monitors. The active sampler uses a personal sampling pump, which is powered by a battery and can be worn either around the waist or in a backpack, to pull air through the media on which the contaminant is collected. Alternatively, the air can be passed by miniaturized sensors, many of which are still under development.

Particles are typically collected on a filter, vapors or gases on an adsorbent, and semivolatile material either using a filter followed by an adsorbent or a denuder (which removes the gas phase) followed by a filter and an adsorbent. The collection media is returned to the laboratory for analyses. Personal sampling pumps operate up to 10 L/min with the flow rate selected based on the duration of the sample and the sensitivity of the detection method with a well-designed study done to optimize the sampling flow rate and duration to be able to detect the contaminant at the level of concern. Passive samples are most often collected for gases and vapors. They use a sampler of a specific geometry to collect contaminants based on the contaminant reaching the collection media due to diffusion and highly efficient absorption of the contaminant. The sampling rate via diffusion is lower than what can be achieved compared to using a sampling pump but has the advantage of being much smaller and lighter than a pump sampler and having no moving parts that could break. Thus, if the concentrations are sufficiently high or sampling duration long, passive samplers are often preferred. The active and passive samplers provide an average or integrated air concentration over the sample duration. Recently, continuous sensors have been developed for various gaseous compounds and for particle counts to continuously measure, store, and/or transmit concentration information for use in an electronic database. These devices provide information on the acute or peak exposure and the average exposure so present advantages for evaluating some types of adverse health outcomes.

For dermal exposure, hand wipes and patches worn on clothing are used to determine the contact an individual's skin could have with contaminants. Hands are the area of the body that has the most contact with surfaces. Hand wipes are collected from both sides of the hands with a premoistened (alcohols, water, or vinegar are commonly used) sampling material that is compatible with the analysis protocol and has low blank levels of the target agent. The hand size should be noted during sample collection. Hand wipes represent what is present on the hand at the time of sampling and often a steady state is established between what goes onto the hand and leaves it from repeated contacts with surfaces. Thus, hand wipes may not represent the total that is absorbed through the skin or may have been ingested through a hand to mouth contact. Patches are placed on parts of the clothing likely to contact agents of concern, such as pants' legs when an individual is walking through or will be kneeling in an area with vegetation that was treated with pesticides.

Food sampling can use the duplicate plate technique where the participant prepares two identical dishes and the portion of food that is consumed on the "duplicate" plate is saved for analysis while the portion that is not eaten by the subject is discarded from the "duplicate" plate. It is important that both the consumed and duplicate plate contained the fully processed food and not just the same raw ingredients as handling and processing of food can change the contaminant loading in the food [38].

REFERENCES

[1] NRC. Human exposure assessment for airborne pollutants: advances and opportunities. Washington, DC: The National Academies Press; 1991.

[2] Ott WR. Development of criteria for siting air monitoring stations. J Air Pollut Control Assoc 1977;27:543−7.

[3] Chen W-J, Weisel C. Concentration changes of halogenated disinfection by-products in a drinking water distribution system. J Am Water Works Assoc 1998;90:151−63.

[4] EPA. US. Integrated review plan for the national ambient air quality standards for particulate matter. Washington, DC: US Environmental Protection Agency; 2008EPA 452/R-08-004, ORD.

[5] Georgopoulos PG, Lioy PJ. From a theoretical framework of human exposure and dose assessment to computational system implementation: the Modeling Environment for Total Risk Studies (MENTOR). J Toxicol Environ Health 2006;9:457−83.

[6] NRC. Exposure science in the 21st century: a vision and a strategy. Washington, DC: The National Academies Press; 2012.

[7] Lioy PJ. Exposure science: a view of the past and milestones for the future. Environ Health Perspect 2010;118:1081−90.

[8] Ott W, Steinemann AC, Wallace LA. Exposure analysis. Boca Raton, FL: CRC Taylor & Francis; 2007.

[9] Lioy PJ. Assessing total human exposure to contaminants. A multidisciplinary approach. Environ Sci Technol 1990;24:938−45.

[10] Lebowitz M, Lioy P, McKone T, Spengler J, Adgate JL, Bennett D, et al. The necessity of observing children's exposure of contaminants in their real-world environmental settings. 2008.

[11] Lebowitz MD, Quackenboss JJ, Kollander M, Soczek ML, Colome S. The new standard environmental inventory questionnaire for estimation of indoor concentrations. J Air Pollut Control Assoc 1989;39:1411−9.

[12] EPA. US. EPA's stochastic human exposure and dose simulation (sheds) model. Washington, DC: US Environmental Protection Agency; 2012.

[13] Glen G, Smith L, Isaacs K, McCurdy T, Langstaff J. A new method of longitudinal diary assembly for human exposure modeling. J Expo Sci Environ Epidemiol 2008;18:299−311.

[14] McCurdy T, Glen G, Smith L, Lakkadi Y. The national exposure research laboratory's consolidated human activity database. J Expo Anal Environ Epidemiol 2000;10:566−78.

[15] Mckone TE. Human exposure to chemicals from multiple media and through multiple pathways—research overview and comments. Risk Anal 1991;11:5−10.

[16] Xue J, Zartarian V, Moya J, Freeman N, Beamer P, Black K, et al. A meta-analysis of children's hand-to-mouth frequeny data for estimating nondietary ingestion exposure. Risk Anal 2007;27:411−20.

[17] NRC. Science and decisions: advancing risk assessment. Washington, DC: The National Academies Press; 2009.

[18] Freeman NC, Jimenez M, Reed KJ, Gurunathan S, Edwards RD, Roy A, et al. Quantitative analysis of children's microactivity patterns: the Minnesota children's pesticide exposure study. J Expo Anal Environ Epidemiol 2001;11:501−9.

[19] Reed KJ, Jimenez M, Freeman NCG, Lioy PJ. Quantification of children's hand and mouthing activities through a videotaping methodology. J Expo Anal Environ Epidemiol 1999;9:513−20.

[20] Zartarian VG, Ferguson AC, Ong CG, Leckie JO. Quantifying videotaped activity patterns: video translation software and training methodologies. J Expo Anal Environ Epidemiol 1997;7:535−42.

[21] Ko S, Schaefer PD, Vicario CM, Binns HJ. Relationships of video assessments of touching and mouthing behaviors during outdoor play in urban residential yards to parental perceptions of child behaviors and blood lead levels. J Expo Sci Environ Epidemiol 2007;17:47−57.

[22] Calabrese F, Colonna M, Lovisolo P, Parata D, Ratti C. Real-time urban monitoring using cell phones: a case study in Rome. IEEE Trans Intell Transp Syst 2011;12:141−51.

[23] Weisel CP. Benzene exposure: an overview of monitoring methods and their findings. Chem Biol Interact 2010;184:58−66.

[24] EPA. US. Exposure factors handbook. Washington, DC: US Environmental Protection Agency; 2011EPA/600/R-09/052F.

[25] Gurunathan S, Robson M, Freeman N, Buckley B, Roy A, Meyer R, et al. Accumulation of chlorpyrifos on residential surfaces and toys accessible to children. Environ Health Perspect 1998;106:9−16.

[26] Morgan MK, Sheldon LS, Croghan CW, Jones PA, Chuang JC, Wilson NK. An observational study of 127 preschool children at their homes and daycare centers in Ohio: environmental pathways to cis- and trans-permethrin exposure. Envrion Res 2007;104:266−74.

[27] NRC. Measuring lead exposure in infants, children, and other sensitive populations. Washington, DC: The National Academies Press; 1993.

[28] Weisel CP, Zhang J, Turpin B, Morandi M, Colome S, Stock TH, et al. Relationship of Indoor, Outdoor and Personal Air (RIOPA) study: study design, methods and quality assurance/control results. J Expo Anal Environ Epidemiol 2005;123−37.

[29] Sexton K, Kleffman DE, Callahan MA. An introduction to the National Human Exposure Assessment Survey (NHEXAS) and related phase I field studies. J Expo Anal Environ Epidemiol 1995;5:229−32.

[30] Weisel CP, Weiss SH, Tasslimi A, Alimokhtari S, Belby K. Development of a Web-based questionnaire to collect exposure and symptom data in children and adolescents with asthma. Ann Allergy Asthma Immunol 2008;100:112−9.

[31] CDC. Third national report on human exposure to environmental chemicals executive summary. Atlanta, GA: Department of Health and Human Services, Centers for Disease Control and Prevention; 2005.

[32] Barr DB, Wang RY, Needham L. Biologic monitoring of exposure to environmental chemicals throughout the life stages: requirements and issues for consideration for the National Children's Study. Environ Health Perspect 2005;113:1083–91.

[33] Weis BK, Balshaw D, Barr JR, Brown D, Ellisman M, Lioy P, et al. Personalized exposure assessment: promising approaches for human environmental health research. Environ Health Perspect 2005;113:840–8.

[34] Wallace LA, Pellizzari ED, Hartwell TD, Sparacino C, Whitmore R, Sheldon L, et al. The TEAM (Total Exposure Assessment Methodology) study: personal exposures to toxic substances in air, drinking water, and breath of 400 residents of New Jersey, North Carolina, and North Dakota. Environ Res 1987;43:290–307.

[35] Heinrich J, Holscher B, Seiwert M, Carty CL, Merkel G, Schulz C. Nicotine and cotinine in adults' urine: The German Environmental Survey 1998. J Expo Anal Environ Epidemiol 2005;15:74–80.

[36] Hoffmann K, Krause C, Seifert B, Ullrich D. The German Environmental Survey 1990/92 (GerES II): sources of personal exposure to volatile organic compounds. J Expo Anal Environ Epidemiol 2000;10:115–25.

[37] Jantunen MJ, Hanninen O, Katsouyanni K, Knoppel H, Kuenzli N, Lebret E, et al. Air pollution exposure in European cities: The "EXPOLIS" Study. J Expo Anal Environ Epidemiol 1998;8:495–518.

[38] Pellizzari E, Lioy PJ, Quackenboss J, Whitmore R, Clayton A, Freeman N, et al. Population-based exposure measurements in EPA region 5: a phase I field study in support of the National Human Exposure Assessment Survey. J Expo Anal Environ Epidemiol 1995;5:583.

[39] Schreiber JS. An exposure and risk assessment regarding the presence of tetrachlorethene in human breast milk. J Expo Anal Environ Epidemiol 1992;2:15–26.

CHAPTER 6

Source to Exposure to Dose Modeling

The primary goal of exposure science is to link the source to the exposure to the dose, and ultimately the mitigation and prevention of hazardous exposure. The mathematical relationship describing the source to dose is critical to both environmental and occupational health issues. The basic equations developed earlier provide a firm foundation for exposure models and source to dose models and systems and can be used to obtain complete quantitative analyses of the exposures [1−7]. However, there are many levels of exposure model systems or modeling systems.

Equations (2.7) and (2.8) can be used to characterize and even define the contributions from one or more exposure routes, r, that lead to a biologically effective dose. A schematic of the processes and variables that should be considered in the development of simple to complex exposure models is found in Figure 6.1. Each of the components and subcomponents illustrate essential variables and data needed to estimate exposures and doses.

Exposure to dose models require input data on the processes within the environment to determine pollutant transport to and through microenvironments; human activity patterns to determine location and duration of contact; physiological data to determine uptake and distribution of toxicants within the body; and metabolic data to determine biological half-lives and metabolites formed. Ideally, these required data would be available for the individuals or population being modeled. When individualized data are not available, generic data bases are commonly used. Generic values for different populations are available through the EPA exposure factors handbook and other handbooks [8−10]. It is critical to match key aspects of the data selected between the study population and information obtained from the handbook. Typical examples are age, gender, and ethnicity, and where possible region of residence. The generic data do not replace the collection of data for an individual or a population of interest, but can be used to fill in data gaps and improve the estimate of external and

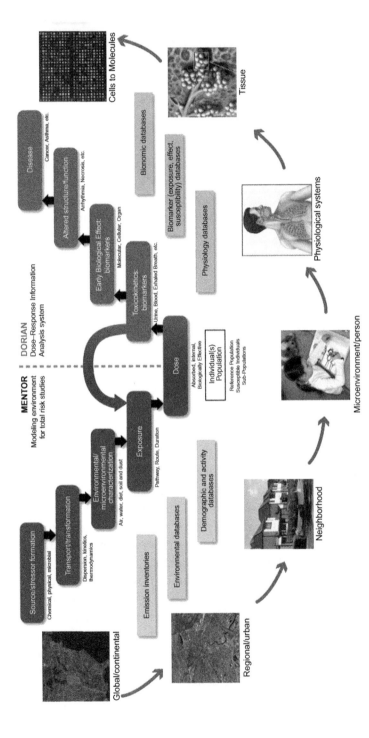

Figure 6.1 *The sequence of processes and scales needed to model human risks due to exposure, using an inhalation example.* Reproduced with permission from Ref. [12].

internal exposures or dose of a toxic agent. They inform the estimate of risk of a disease outcome. The selection of extant data bases requires significant scrutiny since a poor match of attributes of the study population and the generic data can bias the results. Examples of models that rely on extant activity pattern databases to estimate population exposure are the LIFELINETM model which has an emphasis on the dietary route [10], the Stochastic Human Exposure and Dose Simulation (SHEDS) model, a multimedia, multipath way human exposure model [11], and the Modeling Environment for Total Risk (MENTOR) system which is a series of individual and population-based exposure models that are linked to pharmacokinetic models for dose and risk characterization [12]. A comprehensive discussion on the availability and utility of national and state developed extant databases for exposure characterization was published by Lioy et al. (2009) [13].

Well-constructed models can provide full exposure distributions which encompass the mean (average), median (midpoint of distribution), and maximum and minimum exposures to begin to make sense out of the severity of a problem. Statistical methods, e.g., Monte Carlo techniques, have been developed and applied by the US EPA and other government organizations and scientific modifier to estimate distributions of exposure and then the dose for potential long-term and short-term contact with environmental toxicants [11]. These approaches reduce the uncertainty in predicting effects compared to "a single point" estimate.

To summarize the above, a set of seven steps or priorities for examining health outcomes are outlined in Table 6.1 [14].

Table 6.1 Integrated Models for Assessing Exposure and Dose Require Seven Basic Steps

1. Identification of agents, media, and routes of exposure.
2. Identification of target tissue and routes of entry.
3. Identification of the uncertainty in each data base
4. Development of a toxicokinetic model for the agent and the target tissues.
5. Development of a quantitative pharmacodynamics model of the effects caused by the agent in the target tissue.
6. Design of a strategy to collect the appropriate exposure data.
7. Application and validation of models to estimate tissue concentration and exposure index and analyze epidemiological data.

Priorities (Steps) for the health outcomes from doses received by cellular tissue.

The first two steps define the problem to be examined by the model. Steps 3 and 4 define the framework, and step 5 the level of uncertainty associated with the toxicity. Finally, steps 6 and 7 characterize the exposure with new data for the situations of concern and incorporate it into the specific application. A critical component of a model application is an evaluation of the model outputs with measurements, ideally for both the external and internal exposures. The important point to remember is that exposure provides critical information within the source to effect framework. A strength of the exposure model is to predict the potential effectiveness of different approaches to reduce exposure. Depending upon the application, source control or elimination vs. reduction or effective treatment of disease, the collection of new data for use in exposure models can focus on reducing uncertainties in forward or backward applications.

6.1 EXPOSURE MODELS

Exposure models have evolved from models used primarily in the environmental sciences by incorporating human activity patterns to determine contact with environmental toxicants. They have also been expanded to include pharmacokinetic models whose framework was developed for the pharmaceutical industry for estimation of internal exposure and a biologically effective dose. Exposure models have been developed to define population exposures and individual personal exposures. While they borrow tools from other fields to estimate various components of exposure, such as movement of pollutants through the environment, the augmentation of the environmental model outputs with information and mathematical description of human activity, behavior, and physiology was critical to the development of the field of exposure science. The integration of multiple models into a modeling system provides for the transfer of the maximal amount of information among disparate models to improve the source to exposure to dose to disease estimate (Figure 6.1). The focus of the modeling in exposure science is to understand the mechanistic underpinnings of the control of the intensity and duration of contact with a toxic agent.

Many models are available that can simulate the processes and impacts of pollutants in the environment and can provide information on the concentration in a medium over time, the required initial input variables for an exposure model. For example, the strength of the sources of contaminant into different environmental medium can be estimated by emissions models. The transport, transformation, and accumulation parts of the continuum also have many models that explain both physical and chemical processes. Fate and transport models estimate the contaminant concentration at a location for a point in time. However, by themselves, each does not provide estimates of exposure. Models selection should also consider the distance between the source (emissions) and the receptor (population or individual) of concern as near field predictions require different considerations than classic dispersion type models. Exposure models incorporate the above for either an individual or population with information on the activities, behavior, and duration of contact, and are used to estimate the exposure. These results, subsequently, can be linked to pharmacokinetic models for internal dose estimates and pharmacodynamic models for prediction of risk to disease.

One of the first comprehensive exposure models, SHED, was developed by the US EPA [11]. It started as an inhalation model but now can be used for multimedia, multipath way chemicals (SHEDS-Multimedia). It is physically based and evaluates population exposure probabilistically. It can be used in cumulative (multiple chemicals) or aggregate (single chemical, multiple routes) exposures applications to address population exposures associated with the residential and dietary pathways. Recently, SHEDS-Multimedia has been used by EPA to help address US Food Quality Protection Act (FQPA) mandates for registration of pyrethroid, organophosphate, and carbamate pesticides. SHEDS-Multimedia materials, including the accompanying SHEDS-Dietary and SHEDS-Residential modules, are available from the US EPA. Specifically, for user-specified populations, the exposures can be estimated via inhaling contaminated air, touching contaminated surfaces, and ingesting residues from food, drinking water, hand-to-mouth activities, and object-to-mouth activities. The simulations predict ranges of exposure in a population; identify critical pathways, factors, and uncertainties; and enhance dose model estimates. Thus, SHEDS can be used to provide detailed source to exposure estimates for a particular chemical (or group of closely related chemicals) and for a selected route (e.g., inhalation of volatile organics in indoor air or dietary ingestion of pesticide residues in food).

Another user oriented exposure model that has been developed is based upon MENTOR, which is evolving as an open "modeling support system." It is intended to facilitate the multiscale source-to-dose modeling of exposures to contaminants for both individuals and populations. The MENTOR system employs a combination of existing and new modeling approaches to understand environmental and biological processes [4]. To meet the demands for exposure characterization using both extant data and internal and external exposure monitoring data, a new component of the MENTOR system has been developed called PRoT'EG'E (Prioritization/Ranking of Toxic Exposures with Geographic Information Systems (GIS) Extension). It can either characterize or rank exposures based upon the availability of data and the needs of the epidemiologist or risk assessor. PRoTEGE utilizes simplified versions of MENTOR components to provide screening level analyses, employing extant data and modules. It can be used for US-wide (or state/county-specific) simulations of potential population exposures to multiple chemicals for multiple routes and pathway related to all stages of the chemicals' life cycle [15]. It starts with production to usage in various products and to eventual disposal in the environment. The simulations are completed using extant data from standard databases on chemical properties, production, usage, releases, and environmental monitoring networks. This is done in conjunction with "default" distributions of exposure factors for gender and age-defined population segments. This allows "higher throughput" (compared to traditional, case-specific, models such as SHEDS and MENTOR) estimates of population exposure metrics that can support the comparative ranking and prioritization of multiple chemicals, even when available data are limited.

Exposures estimated by the above and other models can be linked to calculate a dose using the pharmacokinetic processes that describe the time-based distribution of the levels of the contaminant or metabolite in the body. Many types of exposure models are described in Refs. [1,12], which discusses the assumptions that must be made for specific applications.

A computationally intensive model that is becoming increasingly important for calculating concentrations distributions of agents emitted by consumer and personal product in occupational settings, homes, other confined indoor spaces, and the center of a city is based upon computational fluid dynamics. These models are used to analyze fluid flows in a confined area which makes them especially useful for problems like street canyons and the flow of air in industrial operations (e.g., clean room hoods). Approximate solutions can be achieved in many cases which should be validated using actual measurements of flow at multiple locations in the study area before being accepted. Ongoing research is expected to yield software that improves the accuracy and speed of complex simulation scenarios such as transonic or turbulent flows. Initial validation of such software is often performed using a wind tunnel that has been set up to replicate the flow conditions being mimicked by the model. They have great utility in estimation of inhalation exposure and can be tested in tracer studies. In the 2005 Urban Dispersion Project for NYC, the US EPA and EOHSI used a task simulation study to provide data on contacts of volunteers walking prescribed paths to simulate realistic exposures of space and time during and after the experiment. The results from this study will be discussed in a subsequent chapter [16].

Other types of exposure models currently being employed use GIS mapping and various regression (e.g., land use regression) and other statistical tools to estimate regional air concentrations for use in exposure models. These approaches have mapped locations of high air pollution and have been used in analyses that estimate large-scale population exposures for ozone and $PM_{2.5}$ [17].

REFERENCES

[1] Duan N. Stochastic microenvironment models for air pollution exposure. J Expo Anal Environ Epidemiol 1991;1:235−57.

[2] Lioy PJ, Smith KR. A discussion of exposure science in the 21st century: a vision and a strategy. Environ Health Perspect 2013;121:405−9.

[3] Henderson R, Bechtold WE, Bond JA, Sun JD. The use of biological markers in toxicology. Crit Rev Toxicol 1989;20:65−82.

[4] Georgopoulos PG, Sasso AF, Isukapalli SS, Lioy PJ, Vallero DA, Okino M, et al. Reconstructing population exposures to environmental chemicals from biomarkers: challenges and opportunities. J Environ Sci Technol 2009;19:149−71.

[5] US EPA. Guidelines for exposure assessment. EPA/600/Z-92/001. Washington, DC: U.S. Environmental Protection, Risk Assessment Forum; 1992.

[6] Georgopoulos PG, Wang SW, Georgopoulos IG, Yonone-Lioy MJ, Lioy PJ. Assessment of human exposure to copper: a case study using the NHEXAS database. J Expo Sci Environ Epidemiol 2006;16:397−409.

[7] Ott WR. Total human exposure—basic concepts, EPA field studies, and future-research needs. J Air Waste Manage 1990;40:966−75.

 [8] US EPA. Exposure factors handbook. EPA/600/R-09/052F. Washington, DC: U.S. Environmental Protection Agency; 2011.

 [9] US EPA. Acute Exposure Guideline Levels (AEGLS) for Chloroacetone (CAS Reg. No.78-95-5). Washington, DC: U.S. Environmental Protection; 2011.

[10] Price PS, Chaisson CF. A conceptual framework for modeling aggregate and cumulative exposures to chemicals. J Expo Anal Environ Epidemiol 2005;15:473−81.

[11] US EPA. EPA's Stochastic Human Exposure and Dose Simulation (SHEDS) model. Washington, DC: U.S. Envrionmental Protection Agency; 2012.

[12] Georgopoulos PG, Lioy PJ. From a theoretical framework of human exposure and dose assessment to computational system implementation: the Modeling Environment for Total Risk Studies (MENTOR). J Toxicol Environ Health 2006;9:457−83.

[13] Lioy PJ, Isukapalli SS, Trasande L, Thorpe L, Dellarco M, Weisel C, et al. Using national and local extant data to characterize environmental exposures in the National Children's Study: Queens County, New York. Environ Health Perspect 2009;117:1494−504.

[14] Lioy PJ. Exposure science: a view of the past and milestones for the future. Environ Health Perspect 2010;118:1081−90.

[15] Georgopoulos PG, Brinkerhoff CJ, Isukapalli S, Dellarco M, Landrigan PJ, Lioy PJ. A tiered framework for risk-relevant characterization and ranking of chemical exposures: Applications to the National Children's Study (NCS). Risk Anal 2014 [in press].

[16] Lioy PJ, Vallero D, Foley G, Georgopoulos P, Heiser J, Watson T, et al. A personal exposure study employing scripted activities and paths in conjunction with atmospheric releases of perfluorocarbon tracers in Manhattan, New York. J Expo Sci Environ Epidemiol 2007;17:409−25.

[17] Maxwell SK, Meliker JR, Goovaerts P. Use of land surface remotely sensed satellite and airborne data for environmental exposure assessment in cancer research. J Expo Sci Environ Epidemiol 2010;20:176−85.

CHAPTER 7

Exposure Science Applications: Within Environmental Health Sciences

Exposure is a key component of both epidemiology and risk assessment but is often estimated at the simplest level which results in exposure misclassification. One reason for this is that large cohorts are studied with little information known about the individuals. In those studies, the exposure characterizations rely on using categorical descriptors of the population for one or more variables across the community, such as the general area that they live in or general industry they work in. A number of reviews of environmental epidemiologic studies have indicated that the exposure characterization is the weak link in their study design [1]. An example of the progression of exposure characterization can be seen for the association of chlorination by-products with cancer and reproductive outcomes. Epidemiologic studies have examined the potential adverse health effects from exposure to compounds formed when drinking water is disinfected with chlorine. Initial studies used an ecological approach to assign exposure based on whether people lived in areas where the water was disinfected (exposed) or areas without water disinfection (nonexposed). However, this approach did not consider whether bottled water or filtered water was consumed and used for cooking, the volume of tap water consumed nor the disinfection status of the water consumed at work or other locations the study population frequented. Further, variations in the actual concentration of disinfection by-products (DBPs) in the water of different subjects were not determined. The next level of exposure assessment incorporated the amount of tap water ingested. Subsequent studies included further refinements to examine other water uses, such as duration and frequency of showering, bathing and swimming to improve estimates of dermal and inhalation exposures. A recent study that incorporated these last refinements identified a gene-environmental association between adverse reproductive outcomes and exposure when the exposure assignment was based on total water usage and exposure [2].

Thus, collection of robust exposure data provides the opportunities for completing exposure–response analyses to reduce to uncertainties and account for confounders and to determine the best approach for risk management and to reduce exposures.

Traditional approaches to incorporate exposure in risk assessment have presented a number of potential problems. First, the exposure assessments can incorporate many invalid assumptions. They included frequent reliance of weak or generic databases which leads to very weak estimations or calculations of external exposure and internal exposure based on uncertain assumptions about contact rates and uptake rates. Risk assessment utilizes the number of grams or milligrams of a toxicant received by the body per day for each route of entry into the body (Table 1.1). When it is applied as part of a site remediation it is often calculated as a screening or baseline risk assessment for multiple exposure pathways and exposure routes. Assessments can be well defined to characterize the risk to the community surrounding the waste site but in some cases the assessment relies on data derived only from samples taken of the waste and on-site media collected during a remedial investigation by a contractor. This latter approach does not provide a comprehensive investigation since that would require off-site media data. The risk assessors use these data to complete screening exposure assessments based upon Environmental Protection Agency (EPA) exposure guidelines [3]. The screening assessment is usually only meant to provide data on the magnitude and extent of contamination, not the extent of exposure. To estimate exposure from these data the contractor typically uses hypothetical individuals completing hypothetical activities in the vicinity of the area under investigation for an estimated amount of time. The hypothetical human receptors can, and usually include: an off-site resident, a commercial worker or business person, a child either swimming in a river or playing on the site, a person completing a recreational activity on site or just off site, such as hunting or fishing. The maximum potential exposure is calculated by assuming a person is actually living on the waste site for many years. As stated previously, these scenarios use a preconceived idea of what people do. The calculated dose is used to identify the major exposure route contributing to the risk.

An additional shortcoming of the above screening approach is that, exposures are applied to individual toxicants rather than mixture of chemicals originating from the waste site. In evaluating the risk from individual toxicants in a mixture it needs to be determined if they are additive which requires that they have the same health end point through the same mode of action [3]. In some cases the mixture can lead to higher risks and in others lower risk. Unfortunately, although the need to assess risk to mixtures has been repeatedly mentioned in the literature it is rarely quantified properly.

Confidence in the risk assessment requires some level of validation in order to reduce uncertainties. The question of study validity is frequently presented during toxic tort proceedings which require statements about the plausibility of an exposure based upon the likelihood that contact occurred. One approach to validate contact is through the use of questionnaire and activity pattern data on the frequency of occurrence of events leading to contact. For example, (1) Did swimming in contaminated waters occur an estimated 2 days per week, or much less? (2) Is it the frequency of eating homegrown foods derived from national databases higher or lower than the consumption in areas of known contamination [3]. Other validations can include measurements using personal air monitoring, tap water samples, shower air samples, dust samples, biomonitoring data, etc. [1]. The unfortunate fact is that current measurements may not reflect the highest historic exposure levels if the site has already been cleaned up or has been provided an interim cap during the remedial investigation. Such information needs to be evaluated for relevance.

7.1 CONFOUNDING FACTORS AFFECTING EXPOSURE

Besides the main variables that describe exposure in epidemiological and risk assessment studies, there usually are additional factors that contribute to adverse health outcomes. These include stressors or confounding factors in the broad categories of genetic, personal, sociological, or economic factors. Factors related to environmental or occupational exposures are presence of polymorphisms, financial status, education level, ethnicity, dietary habits, nutrition, and other behavioral factors. In many epidemiologic studies the target agents are examined in detail but most additional sources and exposures are also not well characterized. One possible exception is cigarette smoking which is known to be a major risk factor for many diseases and therefore generally recorded when personal information or measurements are obtained. Inadequate characterization of the additional exposures can result in bias or in random misclassification of exposures, which when quantifiable is referred to as confounding and can potentially be corrected for in the statistical analysis. Bias misclassification occurs when there is a relationship between the exposure being evaluated and an additional factor. Such an association can result in a differential exposure and health outcome association between the high- and low-exposure subjects. Therefore, unless additional factors are accounted for in the analyses it will not be possible to determine whether the magnitude of the effect seen is due to the target exposure or an additional factor. For example, if all subjects exposed to toluene are also exposed to benzene and those not exposed to toluene are not exposed to benzene then it is impossible to say whether any health effect observed is related to toluene or benzene. If the exposure to benzene is not characterized then health outcomes, such as cancer (which is known to be caused by benzene) could be incorrectly assigned to toluene. When there is no association between the exposure to the target agent and the exposure to an additional factor, any resulting adverse health effects from the additional factor would be randomly distributed across the population. This would result in an increase in the "noise" around the association between the adverse outcome and the exposure to the target agent. Dependent upon the relative magnitude of the adverse effects of the target and additional agents it may not be possible to observe the effect of the target agent unless one can account for confounding factor influence on an observed effect. One of the keys to correcting for influence of other factors that can affect the health outcome is to identify and quantify the plausible exposures and other cofactors and include them in the statistical analyses [4].

7.2 NEW APPROACHES FOR FIELD STUDIES AND SAMPLE ANALYSES ON THE DYNAMICS OF EXPOSURE

A personal exposure study employing scripted activities in conjunction with the release of inert perflourocarbon tracers (PFTs) was completed in Manhattan, New York. Exposures to the tracers were found to depend on many local variables, such as meteorology, traffic, and building geometries along a given route. This novel experiment was conducted as part of the New York Urban Dispersion Program (UDP) that was designed to examine the local horizontal and vertical dispersion of air pollutants released from point sources. The simulated human exposure experiment examined personal contact and exposure to the PFTs in both space and time [5]. The potential exposure patterns were defined through reconnaissance that identified pedestrian and vehicular traffic patterns that might lead to high exposures around the PFT release points. Trained employees completed the scripted tasks. Four different harmless PFTs were released at four separate locations in Midtown Manhattan near Madison Square Garden (MSG) on a sunny day in March 2005. The levels were measured with a variety of stationary monitors located at ground level and in elevated locations. The scripted personal exposure measurements were made simultaneously both during and after the release periods. The personel followed specific paths within an ~5 block area around MSG; each path was associated with common activity patterns (e.g., people evacuating, exiting or approaching the point of release, emergency workers remaining near the release) (Figure 7.1). Each individual wore a passive personal monitor that could detect ppt levels of each PFT and could be operated for a period of time that reflected a 10-min interval of walking time. Lioy et al. [5] developed these scripts based on the information collected by walking the streets and timing exactly how long it took individuals to move through the city at these times of day [5]. The scripted activities were repeated four times to examine the changes in exposure over both space and time of the day.

The exposures were influenced by the surface winds, the urban terrain, and the movements of people and vehicles in urban centers. Typical exposure levels (the higher the vertical bar the higher the exposure) experienced along one route is shown in Figure 7.2. The exposure data indicated that local conditions significantly affected the distribution of each tracer and consequently the exposures and created significant hot spots of PFTs that would not be easily detected by a single stationary monitor. The study provided novel approaches to simulate contacts of individuals with air pollutants and can determine the location of hot spots and potential high exposures. Knowledge about the actual patterns of exposure is useful in the implementation of case control or cohort epidemiologic studies. Scripted exposure studies can be designed around sources of interest and toxic agents or indicator compounds that have well-defined sources and emissions characteristics. These studies would benefit from continuous pollutant sensors to provide better temporal and spatial profiles of the released pollutant.

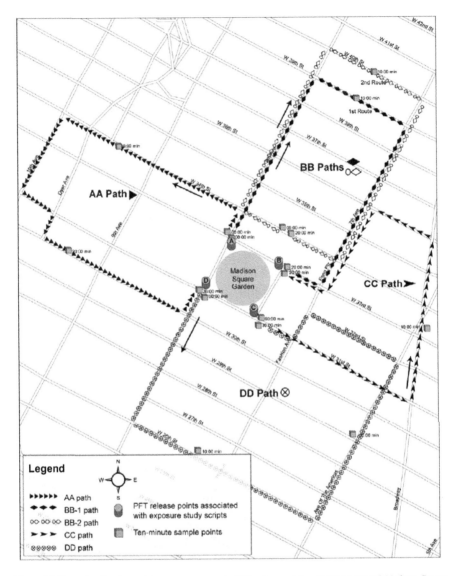

Figure 7.1 The scripted paths used to assess exposure to PFT releases at four locations around Madison Square Garden, NYC. Reproduced with permission from Ref. [5].

7.2.1 GIS, GPS, and Sensors

There are many new tools under development to improve the measurement and characterization of exposure for one or more routes of entry into the body. Some can continuously measure pollutant levels while others track human activity. These will provide insight into acute exposures on timescale of minutes so that peak exposures can be determined.

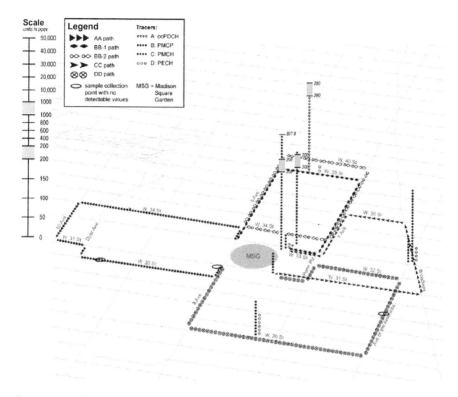

Figure 7.2 Neighborhood scale PFT exposures associated with the scripted paths that examined the impact of PFT releases around Madison Square Garden, NYC. Reproduced with permission from Ref. [5].

Remote sensing technology, including satellite sensors, has been available for a number of years and is being applied to map gaseous and particulate air pollution levels on a population and global scale [1,6]. Mapping of land use and water resources has also been done. Hyperspectral imaging has been used to map pollutants with the appropriate spectral properties that can serve as indicators of toxic agents. These maps provide spatial information and possibly temporal feature of the movement and decay of elimination of materials. Investigators have begun to use personal monitoring sensors to look for a finer scale pattern of contact with some air pollutants and can be used for sub-grid validation of the data collected with mapping data [1].

GPS is being used to track the location of people for a variety of purposes, including safety and surveillance. GPS tracking has great potential for exposure science to continually determine the location of study subjects and potential contact source emissions. GPS has been used successfully in a number of studies with the promise to be able to establish time-based geography of exposure.

GPS data can also be linked to activity diaries to reduce uncertainties in matching locations to activities reported in diaries [7−13]. However, the critical issue is how these data better inform epidemiology and risk management activities. The ability to use GPS to define individualized exposures should improve the characterization of the exposure−response relationship. Similarly, GIS mapping has begun to provide geo-spatial data to map roadways, topographical and urbanization features, population density, bodies of water, point sources and area sources, and roadways and traffic. Some of these maps can be overlaid to develop hypotheses about where differential exposures exist. The drawback of GIS is that data are not real time in most circumstances which prevents establishing time course relationships. There are historical photographs available online which can be examined in parallel with GIS mapping tools to look at long-term changes in any or all of the above.

7.3 WTC AND EMERGENCY RESPONSE/MILITARY

The attack on the World Trade Center (WTC) on 9-11 reminded the environmental health world about acute exposures. Adverse health outcomes from acute exposures were commonplace in the 1950s, e.g., the London smog and Pittsburgh, PA [35]. Even though WTC resulted in an acute event, it was associated with a different category of exposure caused by a terrorist attack. There have been others, with two examples being the Sarin attack of the Tokyo Subway, and the use of mustard gas during World War I. The attack on the WTC, however, illustrated weaknesses in our ability to characterize exposure. Figure 1.1 demonstrated a process needed for going from source to health effect, starting with the source. Though the WTC sources and emissions were easy to identify, they were complex. Two commercial airplanes fully loaded with jet fuel impacted the towers and causing them to collapse. During the collapse millions of tons of concrete and other building materials, furnishings, personal/work items and occupants that were in the interior of buildings turned to dust, and on September 11−12, 2001, an intense fire raged out of control. During the initial response, the need to employ air sampling to immediately characterize the emissions was considered a low priority. Further, traditional air sampling devices would have been useless given the intensity of the emissions and the lack of electrical power. Thus, there were very few environmental or exposure measurements made in the days after the attack. Conversely, there were many individuals being exposed to dust and smoke emitted by the material burned or being resuspended in the area from contaminated surfaces. Among the first monitoring results obtained were for asbestos which in hindsight was not the agent of most concern from an acute exposure [14]. WTC dust samples were eventually taken by the United States Geological Survey (USGS), Environmental and Occupational Health Sciences Institute (EOHSI), and New York University (NYU). The goal was to determine what was in the dust and then determine if there was any need to be concerned that the acute or long-term contact could lead to health risks—the forward approach to exposure characterization—the left side of the continuum [15–17].

The results of the analyses were unusual. The mass was dominated by very large particles (>95%), the pH of the mass was above 9 (caustic); and the dust was dominated by glass fibers, cement and slag wool, and other common materials (Table 5) [15]. Thus, it was not a typical dust nor did it have a typical particle size distribution, with most particles being greater than 10 mm in diameter. A point which would actually be used to understand an evolving health crisis, but at the time did not change the monitoring strategy during the months that followed which was limited to measuring fine particulate matter, $PM_{2.5}$. Then similar to the work of many other physicians during past acute exposure events, physicians, including David Prezant, New York Fire Department (NYFD) and staff at Mount Sinai School of Medicine, identified what would eventually be named the WTC cough. It occurred most prominently in emergency workers who arrived within the first 1–2 days post attack and did not wear any respiratory protection. Thus, the right side of the continuum, Figure 1.1, began to acquire clinical and work activity status information. An acute health response could be expected since the highest exposures would have occurred during the first few days. Eventually, the left and the right side of the continuum reached the bridge, exposure science. It was determined that the WTC cough was most probably caused by the upper airways being irritated by an acute exposure to caustic large particles, glass fibers, and high concentrations of unidentified gases [18,19]. The biomonitoring data from the NYFD was useful in eliminating agents of concern rather than identifying the exposures of interest based on the absence of typical toxic agents or their metabolites in specimens (e.g., mercury) [18].

Today, the measurement of community exposure is still not routinely part of emergency responses, but at least many police officers have portable and real-time radiation monitors due to fear of the use of dirty radiation bombs. Mathematical models for defining when and characterizing what exposure strategies should be employed during what has been described as the 5R periods post a catastrophic event have been developed by Vallero and Lioy [20]. Further, the military has begun to see the need for exposure characterization in noncombat situations [1,21]. The development of new external sensors, and biomonitoring programs, external and internal markers should enhance these efforts.

7.4 DRINKING WATER

Clean water for drinking, personal hygiene, and household uses is critical for maintaining good health. Providing clean tap water to homes requires either a source of pure water, typically ground water, or treating water to purify it, particularly to eliminate microbes. Treatment is common for surface water sources, the predominant water source in the United States and many developed nations. Treatment typically requires a chemical disinfectant to reduce microbial contamination. The most common disinfectants are chlorine based and besides killing microbes result in the oxidation of organic matter in the source water producing DBPs which present their own health risk [22]. Risk assessment is therefore needed to balance the risk from exposure to the biological and chemical agents in drinking water. Chemical contamination (e.g., arsenic in Asia, industrial dumping) and radioactive agents from natural mineral formations and anthropogenic sources can contaminate source water. A key component in determining the risk to contaminants in tap water is characterizing the exposures to those agents. This requires understanding the spatial and temporal variability of the chemical and biological agents within a water distribution system, at the home tap, how tap water is used and the activity patterns of people within residences where others are using water. Water is consumed (ingestion exposure), washed/bathed with (dermal and inhalation exposures), heated releasing volatile contaminants (inhalation exposure) and aerosolized (inhalation exposure). If one returns to Figure 1.1, the source is the purveyor of the water. This can be a municipal water supply or a private well.

Exposure estimates to contaminants in drinking water used to protect public health and in epidemiologic studies have varied from a simplistic characterization of the exposure based on whether a community's water supply relied on routine monitoring results of regulated chemical and biological agents to detailed modeling of water distribution system flow along with measurements of water concentration levels in the system combined with utilization of water and activity pattern characterization of individuals evaluated with biomarker measurements [23]. In determining the exposure to waterborne contaminants the potential exposure routes need to be established for the population and agent of concern. Tap water consumption varies across populations (the young have higher ingestion rates per body mass), location (living in hot/dry climates increase liquid intake), and level of activity (exertion increases liquid intake), pregnancy/lactation, and age. Tap water can be filtered or bottled water can be consumed, which can reduce the contaminant levels, but tap water can also be used in food, flavored drinks, and hot beverage preparation so limiting the ingestion exposure estimate to drinking only plain tap water can underestimate the exposure. Water uses (e.g., showering, bathing, washing, dishwashers, washing machines, toilet flushing, and humidifiers) can release volatile and nonvolatile contaminants into the indoor air of a home [24,25]. The highest exposures will be to individuals in closest proximity to those releases. This exposure pathway is important for volatile compounds, with the degree of release related to its Henry's Law constant which describes the partitioning of a compound between a water and air phase. Under specialized cases, nonvolatile species can become aerosolized contributing to the exposure, but most dose estimates have suggested that ingestion is the more important exposure route for nonvolatile water contaminants. Aerosolized water droplets could be important for respiratory infectious agents in the water supply since exposure to a single microbe can cause illness, though this is not common. Since tap water is used for bathing and showering, dermal absorption occurs for compounds that are lipophilic. The degree of dermal absorption could be altered by use of surfactants in soaps and shampoos [26].

Water contaminants are diverse and can enter the water at the source (e.g., arsenic, radon, pathogenic microorganisms, anthropogenic chemicals such as solvents and gasoline), within the distribution system (e.g., DBPs) or from the plumbing within a home (e.g., lead, cadmium). It is therefore important to understand which process(es) controls the concentration for the contaminant of interest when ascribing an exposure to an individual or population. A new concern is the increasing levels of discarded pharmaceuticals which may be affecting the ecosystem. As their levels in ground water rise they may become an important exposure during pregnancy and for infants whose formulas are prepared using tap water. The introduction of chlorine to disinfect essentially all major municipal water supplies that rely on surface water sources has been a major public health benefit in reducing waterborne diseases but also results in the formation of DBPs, which include teratogenic and carcinogenic compounds. It is necessary to continue to evaluate exposure to pathogenic microbes to assure that resistant species do not develop and adequate disinfection is done to balance the risk between biological and chemical exposures. Two major classes of DBPs, trihalomethanes, and haloacetic acids have been regulated and their multiroute exposures evaluated through monitoring, modeling, and biomarker measurements. Since we must maintain disinfection capability until the water is delivered to the home a disinfectant residual is maintained in the distribution system. Thus, DBPs continue to be produced throughout the water system and within the home in water heaters resulting in variable exposures to individuals within a single water supply system. The DBP levels vary seasonally as the amount of disinfectant required changes with organic load in the source water. To meet regulations and reduce exposures to the regulated classes of DBPs changes to the disinfectant have been attempted. However, alternate disinfectants produce different by-products, may not provide a residual disinfectant capacity (e.g., ozone) or may cause leaching of lead from the pipes if the pH is altered.

Internal exposure measurements of DBPs and their metabolites in blood, breath, and urine along with water concentration measurement can be used to determine exposure in exposure models in order to understand long-term and acute exposure situations. Understanding how and where the individuals actually use water and incorporating differences in metabolism or genetic susceptibility should be coupled with exposure when evaluating risks to individuals and populations, or designing epidemiologic studies.

7.5 THE EXPOSOME AS A COMPONENT OF EXPOSURE SCIENCE FOR RISK ASSESSMENT

The evolution of the field of exposure science has created opportunities to reduce uncertainties in establishing source to outcome relationships for toxic agents. This has led to the introduction of new subareas areas of investigation within the conceptual framework, Figure 1.1. One notable addition has been a concept called the "Exposome." It was first introduced in 2005 by Wild [27] as a complement to the genome.

According to Wild, the Exposome can be defined as encompassing life-course environmental exposures (including lifestyle factors) from prenatal period forward. This concept can include exposures that result from environmental and occupational sources and internal markers of health effects (inflammation and infections) [28]. The approach focuses primarily on the right half of Figure 1.1 and includes measurements to characterize each person's Exposome. The Exposome has been described by Rappaport as a "top-down" approach for addressing environmental and occupational disease. A major goal is to employ "-omic" methods to measure components of human exposure in biological samples. New technology is making the measurements possible, but well-defined, quantifiable -omic markers and improves interpretation of data. Approaches need to be developed that recognize (1) biological markers of internal exposure are highly variable and dynamic as an individual ages and experiences new exposures, (2) health effects will vary across individuals due to genetic differences, (3) the role of single compound versus multiple compounds, and (4) chronic exposures as well as acute exposures need to be considered. The thought is that -omic profiles can be used to generate hypotheses that:

1. Identify specific or series of particular exposures that affect the health of an individual.
2. Develop specific biomarkers for high-throughput screens.
3. Determine sources of external and internal exposure.

Curiously, an external exposure, point 3, is clearly outside of the current scope and capabilities of -omic technology. As illustrated by the continuum, Figure 1.1, external exposure measurements, the left-hand side of the continuum, are needed to successfully test hypotheses. The future effectiveness and utility of the Exposome concept will require an integration of the "bottom-up approach" (external

exposure) with the "top-down approach" (internal exposure) to understand and reduce exposures. Any substantial advances will require validation across both external and internal markers [29]. In a recent
commentary Brunekreef [30] states that "public health will benefit
most when exposure science can help identify which external and internal markers matter most," and can be used successfully to intervene
and mitigate such exposures to an individual and prevent them from
occurring in others.

Exposure science continues to develop the experimental tools necessary to validate and standardize -omic methods in order to combine
external markers (e.g., sensors) and internal markers (e.g., contaminant
and metabolite levels). There are positive steps being taken, including
a focus on approaches to conduct Environment Wide Association
Studies (EWAS). They focus on epidemiological searches for environmental factors associated with disease. The availability of a "chip" or
standard bioassays, which can broadly survey these factors, can be
used to test hypotheses that create a model to assess the influence of
environmental factors associated with disease on a broad scale. EWAS
complements Gene Wide Association Studies (GWAS) which used the
information from the genome project to focus epidemiology on
the genetic determinants of disease. Both are needed to understand the
variability in diseases since the cause of most diseases include environmental and genetic components [31]. The question that needs to be
answered, according to Wild is: can "new "-omic" technology of tran-
scriptomics, proteomics, and metabonomics help unlock problems of
environmental exposure assessment?" [31]. He indicates that the utility
will be proven if altered levels of mRNA, proteins, and metabolites
can be related to specific exposures. Then they will need to be assessed
as to whether or not the results are any more conclusive or accurate
than current techniques that characterize the variability in external or
internal exposure. The approach should include (1) targeted or general
biomarkers, (2) sensor technology, (3) portable and computerized technology (cameras), and (4) improved linkage or internal and external
markers. Fortunately, at some point informatics tools may be able to
help with the integration and interpretation of results obtained with a
wide variety of internal and external markers of exposure.

The field must then focus on the goal of achieving better intervention
and or prevention to reduce disease burden and improve public health.

7.5.1 Summary on Exposome and Exposure Science

If one reviews the Exposome concept carefully, it is actually a rearticulation of the premise of Ott's original idea that exposure is a receptor-oriented science. The key difference is the Exposome, as expressed by Rappaport [32] primarily focuses on biomarker measurements while Ott's concept of receptors is at the external boundaries to the human body [33]. Both embraced the concept of total exposure, with the Exposome considering all routes over a lifetime while Ott's approach recommended examining contact over multiple periods of time and space. A further link between the two approaches, articulated by Lioy [34], is that exposure measurements need to be tied to a biological effect, either acute or chronic, and the time course between an exposure and response or outcome. As emphasized within the continuum, data are needed to bridge our understanding of the relationship between sources and a health outcome. The original proponents of the Exposome have created a very major challenge, since at a minimum to be useful the -omic data require an intense level of information on lifestyle, and behavior. In 2012, Wild [31] revised his initial thoughts on the Exposome by indicating the need for expanded metrics, but proposed using questionnaires to meet this need. Exposure science studies have found questionnaires alone to be insufficient for sustaining real problem solving. Rather the promise of the Exposome can be achieved through studies that link internal and external markers of exposure at multiple levels.

REFERENCES

[1] NRC. Exposure science in the 21st century: a vision and a strategy. Washington, DC: The National Academies Press; 2012.

[2] Villanueva CM, Cantor KP, Grimalt JO, Malats N, Silverman D, Tardon A, et al. Bladder cancer and exposure to water disinfection by-products through ingestion, bathing, showering, and swimming in pools. Am J Epidemiol 2007;165:148−56.

[3] US EPA. Guidelines for exposure assessment. EPA/600/Z-92/001. Washington, DC: US Environmental Protection, Risk Assessment Forum; 1992.

[4] Rothman KJ, Greenland S, Lash TL. Modern epidemiology. 3rd ed. Philadelphia, PA: Lippincott, Williams & Wilkins; 2008.

[5] Lioy PJ, Vallero D, Foley G, Georgopoulos P, Heiser J, Watson T, et al. A personal exposure study employing scripted activities and paths in conjunction with atmospheric releases of perfluorocarbon tracers in Manhattan, New York. J Expo Sci Environ Epidemiol 2007;17:409−25.

[6] Maxwell SK, Meliker JR, Goovaerts P. Use of land surface remotely sensed satellite and airborne data for environmental exposure assessment in cancer research. J Expo Sci Environ Epidemiol 2010;20:176−85.

[7] Calabrese F, Colonna M, Lovisolo P, Parata D, Ratti C. Real-time urban monitoring using cell phones: a case study in Rome. IEEE Trans Intell Trans Syst 2011;12:141−51.

[8] Briggs D. The role of GIS: coping with space (and time) in air pollution exposure assessment. J Toxicol Environ Health 2005;68:1243−61.

[9] Cheng C, Tsow F, Campbell KD, Iglesias R, Forzani E, Nongjian T. A wireless hybrid chemical sensor for detection of environmental volatile organic compounds. IEEE Sens J 2013;13:1748−55.

[10] Elgethun K, Yost MG, Fitzpatrick CT, Nyerges TL, Fenske RA. Comparison of global positioning system (GPS) tracking and parent-report diaries to characterize children's time-location patterns. J Expo Sci Environ Epidemiol 2007;17:196−206.

[11] Engel-Cox JA, Hoff RM, Rogers R, Dimmick F, Rush AC, Szykman JJ, et al. Integrating lidar and satellite optical depth with ambient monitoring for 3-dimensional particulate characterization. Atmos Environ 2006;40:8056−67.

[12] Royster MO, Hilborn ED, Barr D, Carty CL, Rhoney S, Walsh D. A pilot study of global positioning system/geographical information system measurement of residential proximity to agricultural fields and urinary organophosphate metabolite concentrations in toddlers. J Expo Anal Environ Epidemiol 2002;12:433−40.

[13] Schwab M, Terblanche AP, Spengler JD. Self-reported exertion levels on time/activity diaries: application to exposure assessment. J Expo Anal Environ Epidemiol 1991;1:339−56.

[14] US EPA. Mapping the spatial extent of the ground dust/debris from the World Trade Center building. EPA 600/R-03/018. 12/2005, nepis.epa.gov/Exe/ZyPURL.cgi?Dockey=P100BHBE.TXT [accessed 14.10.2013].

[15] Lioy PJ, Weisel CP, Millette JR, Eisenreich S, Vallero D, Offenberg J, et al. Characterization of the dust/smoke aerosol that settled east of the World Trade Center (WTC) in lower Manhattan after the collapse of the WTC 11 September 2001. Environ Health Perspect 2002;110:703−14.

[16] Lioy PJ, Pellizzari E, Prezant D. The World Trade Center aftermath and its effects on health: understanding and learning through human-exposure science. Environ Sci Technol 2006;40:6876−85.

[17] US GAO. Emergency management: observations on DHS's preparedness for catastrophic disasters. GAO-08-868T, 2008.

[18] Prezant DJ, Weiden M, Banauch GI, McGuinness G, Rom WN, Aldrich TK, et al. Cough and bronchial responsiveness in firefighters at the World Trade Center site. N Engl J Med 2002;347:806−15.

[19] Webber MP, Gustave J, Lee R, Niles JK, Kelly K, Cohen HW, et al. Trends in respiratory symptoms of firefighters exposed to the World Trade Center disaster: 2001−2005. Environ Health Perspect 2009;117:975−80.

[20] Vallero D, Lioy PJ. The 5-R's: reliable post-disaster exposure assessment. Leadership Manage Eng 2012;12:247−53.

[21] Lioy PJ. Exposure science for terrorist attacks and theaters of military conflict: minimizing contact with toxicants. Mil Med 2011;176:71−6.

[22] Hrudey SE. Chlorination disinfection by-products, public health risk tradeoffs and me. Water Res 2009;43:2057−92.

[23] Nieuwenhuijsen MJ, Toledano MB, Elliott P. Uptake of chlorination disinfection by-products; a review and a discussion of its implications for exposure assessment in epidemiological studies. J Expo Anal Environ Epidemiol 2000;10:586−99.

[24] Olson DA, Corsi RL. In-home formation and emissions of trihalomethanes: the role of residential dishwashers. J Expo Anal Environ Epidemiol 2004;14:109−19.

[25] Jo WK, Weisel CP, Lioy PJ. Chloroform exposure and the health risk associated with multiple uses of chlorinated tap water. Risk Anal 1990;10:581−5.

[26] Trabaris M, Laskin JD, Weisel CP. Effects of temperature, surfactants and skin location on the dermal penetration of haloacetonitriles and chloral hydrate. J Expo Sci Environ Epidemiol 2012;22:393−7.

[27] Wild CP. Complementing the genome with an "exposome": the outstanding challenge of environmental exposure measurement in molecular epidemiology. Cancer Epidemiol Biomarkers Prev 2005;14:1847−50.

[28] Rappaport SM, Smith MT. Environment and disease risks. Science 2010;330:460−1.

[29] Lioy PJ, Rappaport SM. Exposure science and the exposome: an opportunity for coherence in the environmental health sciences. Environ Health Perspect 2011;119:A466−7.

[30] Brunekreef B. Exposure science, the exposome, and public health. Environ Mol Mutagen. 2013;54:596−8.

[31] Wild CP. The exposome: from concept to utility. Int J Epidemiol 2012;41:24−32.

[32] Rappaport SM. Implications of the exposome for exposure science. J Expo Sci Environ Epidemiol 2011;21:5−9.

[33] Ott W, Steinemann AC, Wallace LA. Exposure analysis. Boca Raton, FL: CRC Taylor & Francis; 2007.

[34] Lioy PJ. Exposure science: a view of the past and milestones for the future. Environ Health Perspect 2010;118:1081−90.

[35] Vallero D. Fundamentals of air pollution. 4th ed. Burlington, MA: Academic Press; 2008.

A.1 GLOSSARY OF COMMON TERMS USED TO EXPRESS EXPOSURE CONCEPTS (ADAPTED AND AUGMENTED FROM [1])

Absorption Barrier   Any surface that may retard the rate of penetration of an agent into a target. Examples of absorption barriers are the skin, respiratory tract lining, and gastrointestinal tract wall (cf. exposure surface).

Activity Pattern Data   Information on human activities used in exposure assessments. These may include a description of the activity, frequency of activity, duration spent performing the activity, and the microenvironment in which the activity occurs.

Acute Exposure   A contact between an agent and a target occurring over a short time, generally less than a day. (Other terms, such as "short-term exposure" and "single dose," are also used.)

Agent   A chemical, biological, or physical entity that contacts a target.

Background Level   The amount of an agent in a medium (e.g., water, soil) that is not attributed to the source(s) under investigation in an exposure assessment. Background level(s) can be naturally occurring or the result of human activities. (Note: natural background is the concentration of an agent in a medium that occurs naturally or is not the result of human activities.)

Bioavailability   The rate and extent to which an agent can be absorbed by an organism and is available for metabolism or interaction with biologically

	significant receptors. Bioavailability involves both release from a medium (if present) and absorption by an organism.
Bounding Estimate	An estimate of exposure, dose, or risk that is higher than that incurred by the person with the highest exposure, dose, or risk in the population being assessed. Bounding estimates are useful in developing statements that exposures, doses, or risks are "not greater than" the estimated value.
Chronic Exposure	A continuous or an intermittent long-term contact between an agent and a target. (Other terms, such as "long-term exposure," are also used.)
Contact Volume	A volume containing the mass of agent that contacts the exposure surface.
Dose Rate	Dose per unit time at the site of action.
Exposure Assessment	The process of estimating or measuring the magnitude, frequency, and duration of exposure to an agent, along with the number and characteristics of the population exposed. Ideally, it describes the sources, pathways, routes, and the uncertainties in the assessment.
Exposure Concentration	The divided by the contact volume or the mass divided by the mass of contact volume depending on the medium.
Exposure Duration	The length of time over which continuous or intermittent contacts occur between an agent and a target. For example, if an individual is in contact with an agent for 10 min a day, for 300 days over a 1-year time period, the exposure duration is 1 year.
Exposure Loading	The exposure mass divided by the exposure surface area. For example, a dermal exposure measurement based on a skin wipe sample, expressed as a mass of residue per skin surface area, is an exposure loading.

Exposure Mass	The amount of agent present in the contact volume. For example, the total mass of residue collected with a skin wipe sample over the entire exposure surface is an exposure mass.
Exposure Model	A conceptual or mathematical representation of the process leading to contact.
Exposure Period	The time of contact between an agent and a target.
Exposure Scenario	Facts, assumptions, and inferences that define a discrete situation for potential contact and exposure. These may include the source, the exposed population, and the time frame of exposure, microenvironment, and activities. Scenarios are often created to aid exposure assessors in estimating exposure.
Exposure Surface	A surface on a target where an agent is present. Examples of outer exposure surfaces include the exterior of an eyeball, the skin surface, and a conceptual surface over the nose and open mouth. Examples of inner exposure surfaces include the gastrointestinal tract, the respiratory tract, and the urinary tract lining. As an exposure surface gets smaller, the limit is an exposure point.
Medium	Air, water, soil, food, and consumer products surrounding or containing an agent.
Pica	A behavior characterized by deliberate ingestion of nonnutritive substances such as soil.
Source	The origin of an agent that releases that agent or provides precursors for chemical transformations that lead to secondary agents that are made available for contact and exposure.
Stressor	Any entity, stimulus, or condition that can modulate normal functions of the organism or induce an adverse response (e.g., agent, lack of food, drought).

Subchronic Exposure	A contact between an agent and a target of intermediate duration between acute and chronic. (Other terms, such as "less-than-lifetime exposure," are also used.)
Target	Any biological entity that receives an exposure or a dose.
Time-Averaged Exposure	The time-integrated exposure divided by the exposure duration but should be relevant to the acute or long-term biological outcome of concern.
Time-Integrated Exposure	The integral of instantaneous contacts over an exposure duration and a concentration of an agent.
Time Profile	A continuous record of instantaneous values over a time period (e.g., exposure, dose, medium intake rate).
Uptake (Absorption or Adsorption)	The process by which an agent crosses an absorption barrier or deposits on a barrier prior to absorption.

REFERENCE

[1] Zartarian V, Bahadori T, McKone TE. Adoption of an offical ISEA glossary. J Exposure Anal Environ Epidemiol 2005;15:1−5.

GENERAL QUESTIONS ON EXPOSURE

1. What are the major variables that affect human exposure beyond the concentration of a contaminant present in a particular medium?
2. Name one of the first individuals to demonstrate a relationship between exposure and human health.
3. How does the bioavailability of a contaminant in a particular medium affect human exposure?
4. What is the difference between aggregate and cumulative exposure?
5. What was the problem associated with the original mathematical expression used to describe exposure? How has this problem been resolved?
6. Give an example of dermal, inhalation, and ingestion exposures that can affect human health.
7. What are some of the challenges to incorporating the concept the "exposome" within exposure science?
8. What is the difference between "microenvironmental" and personal exposure monitoring?
9. How are biomarkers related to internal markers of exposure?
10. What is the difference between external and internal markers of exposure? Why are they both of value in understanding the basic principles and applications of the field?
11. Why is understanding multiroute human exposure important when evaluating lead contamination and emission contribution to children's blood lead levels?
12. What was the first comprehensive study of human exposure, and what was the purpose of that study?
13. What are the primary purposes of human exposure modeling? How has SHEDS been used to understand human exposure issues?
14. What role does house dust play in exposure to semivolatile compounds, such as pesticides?
15. Discuss how proximity to sources affect the relative contribution to exposures?

16. How are questionnaire data used in exposure characterization, and discuss considerations that are used in developing questions to assess exposures?

17. What are some considerations in determining community exposure to toxins from hazardous waste sites?

18. What were the major lessons that you learned about the science of exposure from this book, and how will it improve your ability to solve human environmental health problems?

INDEX

Printed and bound by CPI Group (UK) Ltd, Croydon, CR0 4YY

03/10/2024

01040423-0007